Smart But Feeling Dumb

Smart But Feeling Dumb

Harold N. Levinson, M.D.

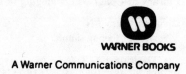

WARNER BOOKS

A Warner Communications Company

The 3-D Optical Scanner, the 3-D Auditory Scanner, the 3-D Tactile Scanner, and the 3-D Visual Trainer are patented.

Warner Books, Inc., 666 Fifth Avenue, New York, NY 10103

A Warner Communications Company

Printed in the United States of America

First printing: November 1984

10 9 8 7 6 5 4 3 2 1

Library of Congress Cataloging in Publication Data

Levinson, Harold N.
  Smart but feeling dumb.

  1. Dyslexia.   I. Title.
RC394.26L48   1984   616.85′53   84-40090
ISBN 0-446-51307-5

Smart but Feeling Dumb is dedicated to:
My dyslexic children
My dyslexic patients
40 million dyslexic Americans
20 percent of the world's population.

Science is an electron in search of its orbit;
Theory is one of many orbits;
Fact is fiction in perspective;
The end is just a new beginning. . . .

I hope the knowledge and insights gained from *Smart but Feeling Dumb* will be the means for a new beginning for dyslexics all over the world.

A dyslexic girl's simplistically composed poem symbolizes the tragic essence and frustration characterizing this highly misdiagnosed and misunderstood scrambling disorder.

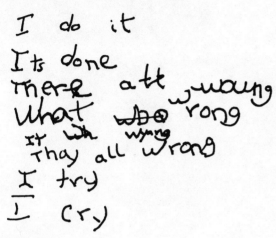

Handwritten by Karen Van Ettinger, age twenty-three, just prior to treatment

Following successful treatment just prior to college graduation, Karen rewrote her poem as she originally intended it to read—clearly highlighting her new beginning.

I do it
It's done
They're all wrong

I try
I cry
They're all wrong

Whats wrong?
Its wrong
They're all wrong.

Table of Contents

Acknowledgments

The basis and focus of *Smart but Feeling Dumb* is the presentation of real, live, currently treated dyslexics, both children and adults. Inasmuch as most of my patients and their families enthusiastically volunteered not only descriptions of symptoms, treatment responses, and their many frustrations in finding meaningful help, but also the use of their true names and circumstances, I feel compelled to credit them for the creation and essence of this book.

My patients and their families did not donate their time, efforts, and identities merely for the sake of acknowledgment. Rather, they wanted all readers to really know what dyslexia and dyslexics are all about. Most important, they want to spare current and future dyslexics the pain, confusion, and frustration that they themselves experienced in attempting to understand and find a solution to this puzzling and confusing disorder.

Smart but Feeling Dumb represents the current scientific reality of dyslexia. If readers—patients, parents, educators, and clinicians—are willing to learn from the insights described within this text, a new era of hope, enlightenment, and success awaits all dyslexics and all involved with the diagnosis and treatment of the learning-disabled.

Several people deserve special mention. Judy Scharle's experiences as a mother of a dyslexic girl led her to write Chapter V, "Trust Me, Sunshine, I'll Find You Help!" Chapter VI, "Determination," was motivated by the incredibly frustrating and inhumane experiences encountered by Dr. and Mrs. "Stone" in attempting to find help for their dyslexic son. Sad to say, they justifiably feared using their real name lest their child be penalized by the educational powers that be. I hope this incredible but true story will lead to the demise and reshaping of these ignorant, egotistical powers. And Mrs. Brody must be credited with her description of her daughter's newfound ability to hear and read as described in Chapter VII, "A Deaf Girl Can Hear Clearly."

Last but not least, I would like to thank my entire staff for their dedicated and untiring efforts in seeing this book to fruition: Grace Gabriel, Joyce Baron, Selma Henick, and Mary Lee. Grace helped collate, summarize, rewrite, and type the clinical content in this book; Joyce helped type and retype the manuscript; Selma and Mary helped organize and maintain my Medical Dyslexic Treatment Center's operation.

I would also like to thank my clinical assistants and technicians; their inner-ear testing was crucial to my formulating an accurate diagnosis and a successful treatment plan.

All the contributors—the acknowledged and the unacknowledged—share one and only one group of common aims:

- To let the insights provided by this work result in a new and successful era for the understanding, diagnosis, and treatment of all dyslexics and all the learning-disabled

- To let no current or future dyslexic continue to feel stupid, dumb, and ugly

- To let no "clinical-educational monopoly" survive that plays and thrives upon the ignorance and suffering of fellow human beings.

Preface

Does your child, student, or patient have a learning problem? Is he or she smart but feeling dumb?

If one or more of the following symptoms are evident, dyslexia may be present:

Reading

- Memory instability for letters, words, or numbers
- A tendency to skip over or scramble letters, words, and sentences
- A poor, slow, fatiguing reading ability prone to compensatory head tilting, near-far focusing, and finger pointing
- Reversal of letters such as *b* and *d*, words such as *saw* and *was,* and numbers such as *6* and *9* or *16* and *61.*

Writing

- Messy, poorly angulated, or drifting handwriting prone to size, spacing, and letter-sequencing errors.

Spelling, Math, Memory, and Grammar

- Memory instability for spelling, grammar, math, names, dates, and lists, or sequences such as the alphabet, the days of the week and months of the year, and directions.

Speech

- Speech disorders such as slurring, stuttering, minor articulation errors, poor word recall, and auditory-input and motor-output speech lags.

Direction

- Right/left and related directional uncertainty.

Time

- Delay in learning to tell time.

Concentration and Activity

- Impaired concentration, distractibility, hyperactivity, or overactivity
- Behavior, temper, or impulse disturbances.

Balance and Coordination

- Difficulties with balance and coordination functions, i.e., walking, running, skipping, hopping, tying shoelaces, and buttoning buttons.

Phobias and Related Mental Disorders

- Fears of the dark, heights, getting lost, going to school
- Fear or the avoidance of various balance, coordination, sports, and motion-related activities
- Mood disturbances
- Obsessions and compulsions.

Did you have academic problems or dyslexia as a child? Do you have phobias and related psychological and physical symptoms that have thus far defied a clear understanding and successful treatment?

- Are you frightened by heights, cars, planes, bridges, elevators, subways, tunnels, open spaces, crowds, department stores, getting lost, losing control, and/or going crazy?
- Do irresistible, repetitive thoughts and actions, obsessive and compulsive actions, harass you and rigidify your ability to relax freely?
- Are you compelled to touch and retouch, check and recheck, think and rethink, and forever make lists of what must be done to avoid memory uncertainty and related anxiety?
- Are you prone to indecisiveness and feelings of inferiority, stupidity, ugliness, and clumsiness?
- Have headaches, stomachaches, nausea, excessive fatigue, concentration

and memory difficulties, or related "psychosomatic" symptoms sent you from medical pillar to post, without avail?
• Are you prone to dizziness or motion sickness?

If any of the above symptoms is present, your phobias and related emotional and physical disturbances may be due to the same *inner-ear dysfunction* as that which I have discovered to cause dyslexia and similar symptoms in children.

As a result of my discoveries, which I consider to be major medical breakthroughs, dyslexia and its related neurotic and psychosomatic symptoms may now in most instances be successfully diagnosed and medically treated. And the inevitable emotional scarring resulting from the dyslexic disorder and its wide-ranging symptomatic fallout can now be prevented or dramatically lessened. At the very least, complex, lengthy, and frustrating psychiatric, neurological, educational, optometric, and occupational therapies have been rendered significantly more successful.

Toward the dissemination of this unique information and understanding—and the early implementation of new and invaluable life-saving medical diagnostic/treatment methods for *all* dyslexics—*Smart but Feeling Dumb* was written.

Harold N. Levinson, M.D.
Clinical Associate Professor of Psychiatry
New York University Medical Center

1

Introduction
and Overview

DYSLEXIA IS COMMONLY RECOGNIZED AS A LEARNING DIS-
order characterized by reading, writing, and spelling reversals. Despite
the growing attention this elusive disorder has received since it was first
recognized in 1896 by two English physicians, J. Kerr and W. P. Morgan,
dyslexia has remained a scientific enigma, defying most attempts at medical understanding, diagnosis, prediction, treatment, and prevention.

Researchers and clinicians were unable to comprehend and define the
dyslexic disorder—unable to understand its wide range of fluctuating
educational, medical, mental, and emotional symptoms—as briefly summarized in the Preface.

Clinicians and educators were incapable of simply explaining to patients
and their families the various underlying mechanisms affecting reading,
writing, spelling, math, memory, speech, direction, grammar, concentration, behavior, balance, and coordination. Few, if any, recognized
fully the depths to which this disorder penetrated the very soul of its
victims. Dyslexia was naively viewed as if it were merely a severe reading
disorder characterized by a fascinating array of reversals. Not recognized
was the agony, suffering, humiliation, and despair experienced by patients
and their families.

- Not recognized was the fact that dyslexics frequently compensate, thus
becoming normal or superior readers, and that a variety of educational, psychological, and IQ test scores could not diagnose or rule out this disorder.

1

• Not recognized was the fact that dyslexia could be a consequence of ear infections, mononucleosis, post-concussion syndromes, or multiple sclerosis.
• Not recognized was the fact that dyslexia may be associated with a wide range of more serious surface disorders, such as mental retardation, cerebral palsy, and deafness.
• Not recognized was the fact that the hidden dyslexic component of the above disorders could be effectively treated for the first time, resulting in an overall improvement in both the hidden and surface disorder.
• Not recognized was the fact that almost all the previously existing assumptions and convictions pertaining to this disorder were found to be in error.
• Not recognized was the fact that most phobias and many so-called mental, emotional, and psychosomatic disturbances were caused by the same physical disturbance underlying and causing dyslexia.
• Not recognized was the fact that many so-called Freudian slips were really dyslexic slips.
• Not recognized was the fact that no traditionally accepted theories and concepts of dyslexia had ever been scientifically validated.
• Not recognized was the fact that no theory could explain and encompass the improvements resulting from all other theoretical approaches: optometric, occupational, educational, psychological, chiropractic and temperomandibular-joint (TMJ), allergic, and nutrition therapies.

In my medical text *A Solution to the Riddle Dyslexia,* I provided the scientific basis needed to comprehend fully and explain the mechanisms and symptoms characterizing this disorder. Moreover, I provided the insights leading to the first medical means of diagnosis, treatment, and prevention, as well as medically determined educational techniques. However, that book was highly technical, and only the most determined readers worked their way through it. Yet, its complexity did not stop many readers; it merely slowed them down. In fact, the difficulty readers experienced with that reading process may be compared to that of dyslexics attempting to read ordinary material: The resulting frustration stops some but not all. For many, the difficulty of *A Solution* merely served to steel their determination to succeed, and a surprising number completed the book from cover to cover—with dictionaries in hand. Many dyslexics and their family members fully digested that technical treatise with voracity and interest, shaming many an expert. However, a simplified version of that text was needed. Crucial insights and medical-educational breakthroughs had to be shared with those afflicted and those interested in helping the afflicted.

With that aim in mind, I undertook the writing of a new book. However, I wanted this new book to contain additional case material and concepts.

Accordingly, *all new case material* has been carefully selected and presented, with the exception of one case which was published earlier, in order to link the old book symbolically with the new.

In *Smart but Feeling Dumb*, I felt the need to highlight the multidimensional nature and complexity of the dyslexic disorder. The common misconception that dyslexia is merely a severe reading or learning disorder characterized by reversals had to be exposed. Clinicians and educators had to be informed that this disorder was as serious and as traumatizing as diabetes, hypertension, and heart disease.

Many educators and clinicians often overlooked and/or denied the disorder's presence and would use such poorly understood diagnostic labels as *stupid, lazy, spoiled, immature, undisciplined, bad,* and even *retarded*. The use of these terms emphasized the underlying presence of "professional" frustration and ignorance. And use of such treatment techniques as scolding, name calling, and "conditioning" merely added insult to injury. Having no alternative and out of desperation, well-intentioned educators and clinicians often encouraged their patients to exercise increased amounts of willpower and determination—as if dyslexics were not already using these functions to capacity—generally with little success.

To highlight and symbolize the emotional and mental depth as well as the scope of the dyslexic disorder, I chose to use a title that emphasized the feelings underlying and characterizing dyslexia. I hope the title and content of this book will trigger the understanding and empathy needed to inspire the interested parent and professional to seek and implement early diagnosis and treatment.

Twenty years of research into the nature of dyslexia, and the analysis of over ten thousand cases, have led me to conclude that most dyslexics feel dumb, despite being smart; hence the title *Smart but Feeling Dumb*. Most often a dyslexic's compulsion to succeed is motivated by an overwhelming desire to prove to himself and others that he is not really as stupid as he feels. Accordingly, the dyslexic disorder frequently serves as a potent stimulus to achieve, reflecting a desperate attempt to reverse the humiliating feelings of inferiority that are invariably present.

Unfortunately, tangible success and peer recognition, even adulation, do not neutralize or eliminate a dyslexic's feeling dumb. All too often, accomplished, even famous, dyslexics merely feel that they have succeeded in fooling everyone around them, and that others are not truly aware of how inept they really are. They attribute their successes to chance, a lucky break, a fluke of nature. Bright dyslexic children who feel dumb invariably become bright adult dyslexics who continue to feel the very same way. Pretty girls feel ugly and handsome boys feel clumsy and klutzy.

Dyslexia does not disappear with age. It is not outgrown. It merely is partially compensated for, which often results in severe emotional scarring. As a result, most dyslexics do not succeed. They do not become famous. They do not overcome. What becomes of them?

Some withdraw or exhibit other antisocial behavior. Most are forced to settle for mediocrity and an inner sense of isolation. Their hopes and aspirations are desperately suppressed, often beyond recovery. Frustration and anger become all-consuming. Many are motivated to direct outwardly their deeply felt feelings of inferiority, inflicting and infecting those about them. Without proper understanding and treatment, the lives of millions of dyslexics are doomed to a continuous stream of failures.

My research has led me to recognize the existence of an unfortunate psychological equation that links dyslexia with feelings of stupidity, ugliness, and klutziness, or lack of coordination—feelings of inadequacy often resulting in social withdrawal, shyness, depression, alcoholism, drug addiction, criminal acts, and years of fruitless psychotherapy. This psychological equation was found to be an intrinsic aspect of the dyslexic disorder in which:

- Feelings of klutziness and clumsiness are derived from the dyscoordination resulting from an underlying inner-ear dysfunction
- Feelings of ugliness are derived from a dyscoordinated, scrambled sensorimotor scheme, resulting in a distorted, "ugly" sense of self, or poor body image
- The disturbances affecting reading, writing, spelling, math, memory, speech, direction, and a host of other related functions result in feelings of stupidity.

The task of writing this book for the layman has not been easy for a medical clinician and researcher. However, an intense need to share my vast clinical experience and success with a greater audience of interested readers has motivated me to compensate for my rather limited writing skills. I hope the content will more than compensate for my rather unique organization and style.

This book was as simply written as I was able. But it is not simplistic or pedantic. It is intended to be thought provoking rather than condescendingly simple. The reader should find it *natural*. By natural I mean that the conclusions will smoothly follow from the case material presented. Complex statistics and scientific design will be avoided, as the scientific background for this book has already been established in *A Solution to the Riddle Dyslexia*.

Most individuals will read this book in order to learn what the symptoms of dyslexia are all about, what positive results can be expected from treatment by a physician, how to best diagnose this disorder early and thereby help their children or themselves to achieve, and how to prevent or minimize emotional scarring. Thus, I decided to write this book in a dyslexialike fashion by presenting the end before the beginning.

Inasmuch as most individuals interested in my research are eager to learn about the patients' symptoms, which define the essence of this disorder, and their responses to my treatment, I decided to present a variety of short case histories right up front. These case histories highlight the disorder and its symptomatic variations at first glance. A sample of individual patient improvements follows, so that the reader may quickly learn the multitude of fascinating responses medications may have.

In viewing the varied case histories as well as the responses to medication, the reader will naturally and intuitively develop a feel for the nature and symptoms underlying and characterizing dyslexia. The many diverse case histories presented will provide the reader with the clinical background needed to judge my research findings independently. Also, by exposing the reader to a large clinical sample, it is anticipated that his understanding will develop as mine did—directly from the patients themselves.

In treating dyslexics both psychiatrically and neurologically over many years, I have come to learn that the only way to neutralize and dissolve their feeling stupid and ugly is to explain to them in honest, straightforward terms exactly what their problems are. They must come to recognize that they have only one relatively simple problem that radiates in a thousand directions, often causing them to feel they have a thousand different disorders and therefore must be crazy and hopeless. In order to feel differently about themselves—to change—they must develop a meaningful insight into the true nature of their problem. They must have a realistic alternative to feeling dumb, ugly, and hopeless.

They must know why they have reading, writing, and spelling difficulties. They must know why and how their reversals and directional disturbances occur, disappear, and even reoccur with fatigue and other conditions. They must truly understand how and why their memory and concentration vary. Dyslexics must fully comprehend why they do poorly in some subjects and well in others. Simply stated, they must understand the essence of their varied dyslexic symptoms to the point of feeling them—a point at which intellectual understanding is transformed into a feeling of conviction, or insight.

With insight, new avenues of approach and compensation will invariably materialize. As a result, dyslexics will develop new ways and means of getting around their problems or working their way through them to a resolution. However, there is one drawback: Someone who thoroughly comprehends the full significance and range of dyslexia must impart this knowledge to the patient and his family.

Inasmuch as I have specifically and thoroughly explained the panoramic nature and cause of dyslexia to thousands of patients and family members, I feel especially qualified to explain this disorder to the reader. I hope you will develop the same understanding as have my many patients and their families.

Patients and their families come into my consultation and diagnostic rooms after an unfortunately long wait. They listen to me and other patients and are amazed at how similar the symptoms of others are to their own despite the many differences and variations that exist among dyslexics. They experience what in psychiatry is called a catharsis. Some are on the verge of tears. They are able to voice their inner emotions and frustrations for the very first time, simply because they have shared them with others with similar backgrounds. Many adults tell me, "You know, I don't really feel *as* stupid or *as* isolated as I did before. I never really told anybody in my whole life how I felt or exactly what symptoms I had."

Following examination of their children, parents are relieved to hear my diagnosis. They have often been previously traumatized with devastating and inappropriate clinical terms such as *minimal brain damage, minimal cerebral dysfunction,* and *mental retardation.* And patients are similarly relieved to find out that they are not just "lazy" or "stupid." Several children have spontaneously asked, "You mean I really have a brain?" Others ask hopefully, "Can I really be helped?" and "Will I be able to play kickball with the other kids?"

In writing *Smart but Feeling Dumb,* I have kept in mind what patients and their families have told me, and I would like to share that information with you. Perhaps you will empathize or identify with their experiences. Accordingly the book contains many variations of case histories, from short vignettes to deep and extensive revelations. You will hear patients convey their agony in dealing with the dyslexic symptoms. You will hear the frustrations and pain of family members, as well as their added suffering when periodically dealing with clinically inexperienced, defensive, sometimes offensive professionals.

The sample case variations have been chosen to facilitate the reader's finding himself in the situations presented, just as my patients and their parents do while they patiently and hopefully chat and listen to others in my waiting room. After assimilating the case histories and the patient responses to the medication, I feel the reader will be ready to grasp naturally both the history and significance of my research efforts—efforts that have led me to resolve the medical diagnostic and therapeutic void in dealing with dyslexia. A typical treatment response as observed by a patient's mother, highlights the meaning and significance conveyed by this introduction and overview—indeed, this book:

> Words can not express the new Karen you have given us! There is a lot of work to be done to help her compensate for the basics she lacks, but with her newfound abilities, we are all optimistic! I feel that you have, indeed, changed our lives to the good! Thanks to you and your staff.

Karen Torgenson is an attractive, extremely articulate, and socially mature young lady of fifteen years. She is also very gifted musically and artistically. However, as the Torgensons relate, it was as though Karen were two girls rather than one. One girl was charming and attractive, with a prodigious capacity for self-discipline in art and music and admired in both areas by her peers and adults.

The other girl was seething with anger, resentment, and frustration with her academic subjects and her teachers. She seemed to have a total block to learning subjects that required reading, concentration, math, memory, and organization. She lacked interest and self-discipline with her homework and school projects other than those pertaining to art and music. This Karen either lashed out bitterly and unreasonably at her family or retreated behind the closed door of her room.

It was very difficult for her parents and others who knew and loved Karen to reconcile these two completely different halves of her character.

All of her life Karen talked in her sleep and sleepwalked three or four nights a week. During these episodes she appeared very pensive, worried, and anxious to either rearrange items in her room or to leave the house, mumbling in an agitated fashion about needing to "fix things" or about some impending crisis. For her parents, both of whom are teachers, the situation was particularly painful. They gave Karen loving support and assistance in studying and completing assignments. Karen's father, who teaches at her school, tried to keep open the lines of communication and understanding between his daughter and her teachers while simultaneously attempting both to encourage and inspire Karen. Needless to say, this task was most difficult and emotionally draining for all.

These were the circumstances in the Torgenson family in October 1982. From friends they heard hopeful and favorable reports about my Medical Dyslexic Treatment Center and the many dyslexics who were being helped. Accordingly, this family came to the center, where Karen was examined and prescribed medication. Eight weeks later, in a progress report, Mrs. Torgenson wrote: "Karen surprisingly stated, 'I don't feel mad anymore!'" Moreover, Karen felt less tension and irritability and her sleepwalking stopped the very first day she was given medication. "I can see an inner composure and tranquillity not previously present," Mrs. Torgenson observed. "She is able to concentrate, to follow through on homework, and to learn new information."

Karen was now accepting and responding to hugs and expressions of love from members of her family. "It had gotten to the point that she would hardly acknowledge a kiss on the cheek," Karen's mother continued. "However, since I think hugs and kisses are indispensable to children of all ages, I continued to seek her out, even though she felt unlovable. Some days it was the only way I could tell her that we loved her in spite of her problems. It is a joy to have her come up and hug me now!

"At home, she is reasonable and more controlled. There are far fewer outbursts of frustration. I sense in Karen a feeling that she is able to take control of her life. She has pride in getting her homework done on her own. She has even seen the English teacher, for example, about how to improve her basic skills, and she is keeping a check, on her own, of all her grades."

Karen's father remarked that one year earlier, Karen's grades were D's and F's, even in below-average-track classes. She skipped some classes and did her homework only under duress. Today, Karen's grades are C's and $C+$'s in regular classes. She no longer skips classes, and on her own initiative she completes her homework on time. "There is still much work to be done—gaps to be filled in . . . but giant steps have been taken toward achieving these goals," Mr. Torgenson says.

Karen's mother related several additional instances that showed clearly the remarkable changes in her daughter's attitude and personality.

The first occurred about six weeks after medication had begun. Karen sat down at the piano to sight-read a song, previously a very frustrating task for her, one accompanied by tenseness in posture, scowls, and many mistakes of which she would not normally be cognizant unless pointed out. On this day, however, she sat down at the piano and approached her task with composure and logic. When she made a mistake, she immediately picked up on it and corrected it on her own. Since I am a piano teacher, I was nothing less than thunderstruck at the improvement that occurred in her.

A second incident occurred a few months later. Karen was working with her sister on a very difficult saxophone solo. Since it was a Saturday, she was off her medication.* She approached the practice irritably and somewhat negatively. As they progressed she became increasingly frustrated and angry with herself because she could not execute the notes as she knew they should have been played. Pretty soon she was stomping her foot and berating herself quite vocally for her "stupidity." I told the girls to take a break and gave Karen her medication. Forty-five minutes later she returned to practice, calm and with no signs of irritability. Karen was amenable to suggestions, concentrating, and working through her difficulties.

Later her sister commented to me about the difference the medication made in Karen's attitude and behavior. The two girls had worked intensively for two hours, and Karen had handled it quite well. Both girls accomplished much during this time.

A third incident occurred one month later. Karen and I were playing tennis. Nothing seemed to go right for her: Either she missed balls or the balls went into the net. She became angry and disgusted with herself. She took her medication, and after a half hour's respite she resumed playing. Karen performed normally and with composure. She occasionally hit a crazy ball, as everyone does, but her feelings and behavior were more appropriate to the situation.

The dichotomy in Karen's personality and performance has become more and more a thing of the past. The Karen whom friends, parents, and teachers now see and deal with is an integrated person who reflects a happier, more self-assured and enthusiastic personality and who eagerly anticipates each day. She has learned to care for and respect herself and, in doing so, has become able to express love and admiration for those closest to her.

Of no small significance is the fact that Karen's feelings of stupidity and inferiority rapidly dissolved as soon as there appeared a positive inner change secondary to the medication. Thus, she could accept her mother's affection and even return it. She no longer felt ugly, stupid, hopeless and "unlovable."

By reading the following case responses, which are similar to Karen's, you will develop a feel for the many symptoms and their variations characterizing dyslexia. In this manner you will be following in my footsteps. I have repeatedly stumbled upon unexpected dyslexic symptoms. Here I have attempted to explain them all, including the sleepwalking.

*I often instruct patients not to take medications on weekends and holidays and over vacations, if possible. This procedure minimizes the chances of becoming "immune" to the medications while it increases the chances for maximum compensation. For more on how dyslexics compensate for their symptoms, see Chapter IX, "The Symptoms and Mechanisms Defining Dyslexia," p. 108 (Author's note).

By realizing that sleepwalking stopped on medication, it became obvious that yet another symptom could be added to the list of dyslexic characteristics, some of which were highlighted in the Preface. In a similar fashion, a whole series of unexpected findings were noted when patients and/or their parents spontaneously reported the changes noted with the medications.

For example, I discovered that many dreams of falling and flying, and even dizzy dreams, are shaped by dyslexic mechanisms. In fact, the rapid eye movements (REMs) used to track dream content are identical to the eye movements and mechanisms utilized by nondyslexics and dyslexics to track letters, words, and numbers. And both inner dream tracking mechanisms and outer word tracking mechanisms may be similarly disordered in dyslexics.

Levels of sleep may be altered by the dyslexic process and the response to medications. Thus, insomnia and sleepwalking may be reversed by restoring the patient to normal levels of alertness and sleep states. Individuals who never dreamed before will suddenly dream and will remember their dreams. And the dream content may even change or become more colorful.

Analyze my patients' responses very carefully. I hope you will find them helpful. Reason out your own inferences and conclusions, and match them to mine. Do not be misled by theories and theorists unless what is said corresponds to the clinical responses reported by dyslexic patients. *Remember, dyslexic patients ultimately define the dyslexic disorder, not experts.*

In retrospect, most of what I have read about dyslexia seems to me to be completely or significantly wrong. Too much written information appeared independent of clinical experience.

By the end of the book I hope sufficient clinical content will have been presented so as to enable you to clearly discern dyslexic fact from fiction.

2
Understanding Dyslexics

THE ONLY WAY REALLY TO UNDERSTAND DYSLEXIA IS TO understand dyslexics. Reading, writing, spelling, and math scores do not really tell you what dyslexia or dyslexics are all about. In fact, these scores are often confusing to readers, parents, and patients—and especially testers. Although some scores are truly needed for educators to begin responsible remediation, I doubt that all the reported scores and numbers are helpful to anyone except the computer and test salesman.

Clinicians, parents, and dyslexics all want to know the same things:

- What symptoms characterize the dyslexic disorder?
- What distinguishes these symptoms and this disorder from other types of learning-related disabilities?
- How can the symptoms and the disorder be most effectively, expediently, and accurately diagnosed and treated medically, educationally, psychologically, optometrically, etc.?

All of these questions will be answered by the time you finish this book. However, this chapter is primarily devoted to answering only the first question. By reading the case histories, you will develop a feel for the *quality* of the dyslexic disorder and its diffuse and varied symptomatic fallout. This quality has never before been clearly recognized and appropriately described. The reason for this failure is tragically simple.

Dyslexics cannot answer questions they have never been asked! They do not specifically and spontaneously relate and describe their many

11

symptoms and feelings to testers only interested in obtaining numbers and scores. And sad to say, quantities and numbers—and the statistical analysis of these numbers—often fail to elucidate the quality and essence of the disorder tested. Indeed, the seemingly infinite variety of tests and scores (what I call the "test and number compulsion") actually masks and further complicates the recognition and definition of the disorder under investigation.

Numbers and scores most certainly have their place in science and research. They are most effective in biological research, especially where the subject tested cannot verbally respond, as in the cases of apes, dogs, and unconscious patients, and in chemical assays. But as scientists we should not rely *entirely* on numbers when attempting to understand the symptoms experienced by human beings who are desperately attempting to verbalize and clarify.

Why not ask these patients what is wrong with them or how they feel? Let them tell you! Record the details in the same meticulous manner you would record their test scores. And when a pattern of symptoms emerges, ask more specific questions in order further to pin down and define this pattern. And behold: Much of the dyslexic disorder will develop and materialize before your eyes!

In other words, where possible, first learn the *quality* and essence of the disorder. Develop a feel for the scope of its symptomatic and variable fallout. Then obtain the needed scores and statistics to highlight and determine more closely the disorder's dimensions.

The numbers that have been used until now to characterize and define what has been commonly referred to as learning disabilities, dyslexia, and developmental delay have not been able to separate one disorder from another or one symptom from another. Indeed, these numbers have led to a dyslexialike scramble and confusion, serving no one except perhaps special-interest groups attempting to hide their own inner frustrations.

Utilizing recorded cases and symptoms, I will sketch a concept of the dyslexic disorder that can explain and encompass every known symptom and mode of therapy characterizing dyslexia to date.

Katie

Katie, you are just too slow! You make the same stupid errors over and over again. Can't you remember the difference between a *b* and a *d* and the words *was* and *saw*?

And you still can't add or subtract correctly without using your fingers. You're not a baby: Don't act like one!

Katie's teacher yelled at her thoughtlessly. A dozen years later, a troubled teen-ager was brought to my office for psychiatric treatment. She could not think or talk about that day without crying.

Not much had changed for Karen over the years. She continued to feel stupid and ugly, despite a superior IQ and a very attractive appearance. She cried, "How smart can I be? I still can't tell my right from my left. I really must be a moron!" Unfortunately she had overheard a noted colleague of mine diagnose her as having "minimal brain damage." "Not only am I stupid, but I am brain-damaged as well. How do you expect a moron to feel?"

Jimmy

- Jimmy couldn't ride a bike, participate in sports, climb a fence, or climb a tree.
- He held a pencil tightly and awkwardly, as though he were holding on for dear life.
- He often lost his balance and fell. He frequently walked into walls and doors or tripped over his feet. Klutzy and Clumsy were his nicknames.
- Reading triggered headaches, dizziness, nausea, and stomachaches.
- Finger-counting enabled him to add and subtract. When older, he would forget the multiplication tables as rapidly as he learned them.
- Jimmy avoided heights and sports. Elevators and escalators panicked him. Amusement rides and flying in planes led to disorientation. New and unfamiliar places made him clinging and fearful of becoming lost.
- Anxiety appeared to trigger bed-wetting.

When Jimmy turned fifteen, he was referred to me for psychiatric treatment because of depressive feelings and suicidal thoughts. When I first asked him what was wrong with him, he stated: "I'm just stupid and klutzy. The school says I have to accept these facts. And one of my teachers even thinks I am retarded. . . . So do I."

Karl

Karl cried continually from the day he was born. He was restless, colicky, and unable to sleep. Repeated examinations found him to be a "normal" infant. When six weeks old, his ears were found to be badly infected and his eardrums bulging, ready to burst. Surgery relieved this pressure. Suddenly gone were his crying, restlessness, and colicky symptoms. He slept peacefully. However, he remained hyperactive.

- Although Karl ran and climbed early, his developed very slowly.
- His words and sentences were poorly articulated and organized, rendering his speech difficult to understand.
- Although sharp and alert, his attention span was short and he was easily distracted.
- Despite normal hearing tests, statements and directions had to be continually repeated, slowly and one at a time.

Kindergarten and first grade intensified Karl's hyperactivity and distractability. Teachers frequently complained that he didn't listen and that he left his seat and roamed around the room. He was forever squirming in his seat or moving about restlessly. At first Karl was ignored. Then he was teased, which provoked him to lose his temper and overturn chairs, desks, or anything else in his way.

Karl could not express or verbalize his feelings and thoughts. He preferred action to speech. Accordingly his acting-out behavior was not really purposely antisocial; it merely reflected an emergency discharge of frustration by a child who could not verbalize what was really bothering and frustrating him.

By first grade Karl refused to attend school. He found it too confusing, frustrating, and humiliating. Psychologists believed him to be suffering from a school phobia and advised his parents that Karl's fear of leaving them was due to their overconcern and overpampering.

- Ignored by clinicians was the fact that Karl did not fear leaving his house.
- Ignored was the fact that Karl did not fear leaving his parents. He merely feared the frustration and confusion triggered by the school situation.
- Overlooked by the school personnel was the fact that Karl could not handle reading, writing, spelling, drawing, and the many distractions of a classroom full of other children.
- Overlooked was the fact that Karl was not truly antisocial. He liked individuals but could only handle one at a time. He was not truly aggressive; he just had difficulty acknowledging and verbalizing his many frustrations.

School phobia was the first of many diagnostic terms used by subsequent clinicians. Karl's diagnoses were everything from school phobia and behavior disorder to minimal brain damage and even congenital aphasia.*

• No one recognized that Karl was dyslexic.
• No one realized that his behavior disturbances were merely part of the hyperactivity and distractibility characterizing the dyslexic syndrome.
• No one knew that the speech disorder he suffered from was a consequence of his dyslexia. It was not an expression of a dysfunction in the thinking brain. It was certainly not aphasia.
• No one appeared to understand that underlying Karl's apparent bravado and "delinquentlike" acts were feelings of intense stupidity.
• No one suspected that these hidden but devastating feelings existed until they suddenly and dramatically materialized during psychiatric treatment.
• No one appeared to acknowledge that early diagnosis and treatment would have saved Karl and his parents a great deal of tragic suffering.

Laura

Laura was a gifted child. She spoke when she was six months old and conversed with adults when she was a year old. She knew her basic skills from watching *Sesame Street*. As a result, she didn't attend kindergarten, breezed through the first and second grades, and captivated everyone with her bright and delightful ways. In the third grade, however, something happened: Laura seemed bored. And during the fourth grade her joy in school seemed to have vanished. She tried to avoid reading and writing assignments and showed no interest in classwork. Psychiatrist friends told her parents that Laura was spoiled, overpampered, overloved, and not sufficiently disciplined.

Laura was diagnosed by me to be dyslexic. Fortunately she responded successfully to medication. Laura regained her curiosity, confidence, and interest in school.

Laura was not the only one to benefit. Laura's parents, who were very much affected by their daughter's suffering, could never have held together as a happy, loving, caring family without a thorough understanding of Laura's symptoms and a way to treat them.

My insight into Laura's condition developed as I considered her symptoms and realized that she:

*Aphasia is a severe speech disorder in which disturbances of the thinking brain result in difficulty understanding the meaning of what is heard and/or difficulty formulating the meaning of words and thoughts one wishes to express.

- Avoided reading because she skipped or reversed letters and words
- Perceived sentences to be slanted and, in order to compensate, used angulated reading postures that are generally considered to be careless or sloppy
- Could not keep her handwriting from drifting off the page because the physical act of writing was dyscoordinated for her
- Frequently tripped and fell
- Turned in "sloppy" homework and kept her bedroom "messy" due to the same factors that resulted in her scrawled handwriting, awkward walking, and propensity for accidents
- Knew right from left only because she had learned at a very young age that she wrote with her right hand and wore her baby ring and watch on her left
- Feared leaving home and going to camp—fears related to her directional uncertainties, the same compass disturbance that earlier had her clinging to her parents and home
- Was susceptible to motion sickness, which in turn resulted in motion-related fears of elevators, escalators, planes, etc.
- Suffered from so-called psychosomatic headaches, dizziness, and abdominal pains—symptoms triggered by motion-sickness mechanisms
- Was very hesitant and reserved with strangers because of her secret feelings of being overwhelmed, uncoordinated, or "klutzy."

To summarize, all Laura's symptoms were intimately related to, and determined by, her dyslexic disorder.

I arrived at my diagnosis of Laura when I discovered a youngster could begin school as a good reader yet still be dyslexic. In other words a dyslexic need not be word-blind and often is not. The reading symptoms in dyslexics often reveal themselves only when there is an increase in the quantity of material to be read and when the print is smaller and closer together than usual, requiring an increase in reading speed and targeting accuracy, all of which happens in third grade.

When diagnosis opened the way to treatment for Laura, I felt that all my efforts, commitment to my work, and years of research had rewarded me in full with the recovery of this one special patient. Laura's case was not the initial impetus for my original studies, but she has been a most important patient, and one of many to benefit from my research. Laura is my daughter.

Joy

Joy mastered the first few years of school effortlessly. But suddenly she developed a paralysis of her limbs due to infectious mononucleosis. She became dizzy. Her concentration became foggy. Fortunately, her paralysis was overcome, but her immunity system had been impaired, which resulted in repeated viral and strep infections, including ear infections. Joy's ability to concentrate lessened and her frustration tolerance decreased. At the same time, her sensations of dizziness and motion sickness intensified. She began to reverse and misplace letters and words when she read, spelled, or wrote. She became disinterested in studying and in school.

Joy's parents were advised by physician friends and teachers that Joy was overloved and indulged as well as manipulative. Whether or not this was true was beside the point. How could parental concern and love create word reversals and other symptoms of dyslexia?

They cannot, of course. The fact that dyslexic symptoms are found to be present in pampered, neglected, and even abused children leads to the important conclusion that the presence of dyslexic symptoms is independent of child-rearing patterns. In fact, I discovered this disorder to be dependent upon hidden physical factors that lie in the inner-ear system.

Understandably, Joy's parents were very concerned. They knew that their daughter's problems were not caused by their concern and love but by repeated ear infections. Joy's difficulties—her impaired concentration, her word reversals—all sprang from middle-ear inflammations or infections that affected her inner-ear system, the system responsible for the fine-tuning and coordination of all sensory input patterns and all body movements.

I placed Joy on medication, which initially led to an improvement in her *acquired* dyslexic symptoms. Also, I suggested that she have her tonsils and adenoids removed, and that draining tubes be placed in her ears, a procedure used to eliminate and prevent fluid accumulation. Happily these surgical procedures successfully eliminated her repeated ear and throat infections.

Joy, too, is my daughter.

Studies I conducted over the last few years clearly indicated that well over 95 percent of similar cases responded to these surgical procedures as well as my daughter did. Unfortunately, many physicians are unwilling to perform these simple surgical procedures, preferring to wait until children "outgrow" their susceptibility to ear infections and tonsilitis. However, too many cases do not outgrow this tendency, just as they do not outgrow their dyslexic tendencies.

What happens while we wait? Children remain vulnerable to repeated and chronic ear and throat infections. They miss school and fall behind in their subjects. They are unable to socialize or participate in sports events. Their immunity systems become increasingly impaired. They develop allergic reactions to antibiotics and other medications. And they are predisposed to permanent hearing loss and/or ear disorders resulting in dizziness, motion sickness, and a host of dyslexic symptoms.

It appears that medical opinions often swing from one extreme to another. When I was a child, all one had to do was open one's mouth for tonsils and adenoids to be removed. Now one practically has to be on one's deathbed before they are taken out. Needless to say, these extremes make no sense.

To return to Joy's case: After her surgery she felt stronger, but this did not last long. Her dizziness returned, as did some of her previous symptoms. In addition, she developed severe, chronic headaches, at times migraines. The medications no longer seemed effective. At first I thought her body had developed an immunity to them, but something else was wrong.

Joy walked in a slumped fashion and appeared depressed. She could not overcome her feeling of fatigue. Her concentration and memory functions dwindled significantly from superior to frighteningly poor. She developed facial, neck, back, and leg muscle spasms.

She developed pain in her ears, which persisted even after the draining tubes were removed. We returned to the ear, nose, and throat doctor, who claimed that the procedures he had performed were successful. Nothing appeared to be wrong with her ears.

Then, one summer, Joy's mysterious symptoms were accidentally diagnosed while she was a junior counselor at camp. She noticed that one of the other counselors missed camp periodically and that this counselor's personality varied from time to time, just as her own did. At times the counselor was "sweet as sugar," and at other times she was irritable.

Joy discovered that the counselor had severe migraines, which were responsible for the fluctuations in her mood and behavior. Upon talking to her, Joy learned that the counselor had temporomandibular joint syndrome (TMJ). Further questioning revealed that the counselor had symptoms identical to her own.

In retrospect I realized that Joy's TMJ syndrome was caused, or significantly intensified, by the clamps that had kept her jaws widely separated during her surgery. It seemed ironic that the surgery needed to save her ears and health had inadvertently resulted in a disorder with symptoms similar to the ones it was intended to alleviate.

In addition, I and the dentist treating her TMJ, independently but simultaneously, realized that Joy also had symptoms suggesting the presence of an underactive thyroid, or hypothyroid, condition. She is currently being treated to correct and compensate for both her TMJ syndrome and thyroid disorder. Many of her symptoms have already been alleviated by means of this multidimensional approach. We hope that all the symptoms will disappear.

Joy's case clearly highlights the fact that dyslexia may be acquired or intensified by mononucleosis or ear infections. Moreover dyslexia, a highly misunderstood and oversimplified disorder, may be complicated by other hidden coexisting disturbances, such as TMJ, thyroid disease, diabetes, and hypoglycemia.

Bonnie

Bonnie was twenty-nine years old when she initially consulted me for severe depressive feelings and phobias—a fear of becoming ill and dying as her mother did, a fear of traveling and new places, and a fear of heights. Also, she had "heard voices" intermittently during her entire life. This symptom had led psychiatrists to misdiagnose her as a schizophrenic.

Bonnie has two children. Following each childbirth her symptoms had intensified so much that she required hospitalization.

I came to realize that Bonnie's depressions, fears of illness and dying, and even her voices were all related to her mother's having died immediately following Bonnie's birth.

Bonnie felt extremely guilty about her mother's death. Her "voices" were found, upon analysis, to be related to her mother's absence. She had always thought about her mother and conversed with her while daydreaming, forever imagining what her mother would say in this situation or that. She could actually hear these daydreams: Bonnie's "voices" reflected her need to regain and maintain contact with her beloved but lost mother.

As stated, Bonnie blamed herself for her mother's death. Had she not been born, she believed, her mother still would have been alive.

Following the birth of each of her children, Bonnie became increasingly depressed, anxious, and fearful. Her conscience became increasingly harsh and intense during these episodes. Clearly, Bonnie was suffering from hysteria, not schizophrenia.*

*Hysteria is a relatively mild and psychoanalytically treatable emotional disorder in which the symptoms are determined by unconscious needs and wishes. By comparison, schizophrenia is a severe emotional disorder of unknown origin and uncertain prognosis.

Upon careful questioning I found Bonnie had been a poor student as a child, had had difficulty reading, writing, and spelling, and had been a stutterer. She also admitted to always having felt stupid and unattractive. The stuttering still persisted, as did her feelings of inferiority. I initially assumed that all of Bonnie's symptoms were emotionally determined and treated them all psychotherapeutically. Her treatment was successful. She eventually raised three children, survived two surgical procedures without emotional relapses, returned to college, and earned master's and Ph.D. degrees. And she no longer felt stupid and ugly.

Only in retrospect did I recognize that Bonnie's early academic and speech difficulties, as well as her fears of heights, elevators, needles, illnesses, new places, and driving, were manifestations of a physically determined inner-ear disorder—dyslexia. I came to realize that her feeling stupid and ugly were as much determined by her dyslexic disorder as by her hysterical disorder. Even her "voices" appeared to have a physical co-determination. Dyslexic children occasionally compensate for their memory disorder by developing eidetic* imagery. Bonnie's voices had had a compensatory eidetic quality.

When I first began treating Bonnie psychotherapeutically, I had not yet recognized the physical basis of her many symptoms. I had been treating her *only* psychiatrically, not physically or holistically. I did not yet appreciate the full significance and wisdom of Sigmund Freud's remark that underlying and co-determining all emotional symptoms is a physical basis. This basis he called "somatic compliance."

Randy

Randy, married and the mother of two children, is a thirty-four-year-old homemaker. She came to see me for psychiatric help because she was subject to mounting fears and anxieties.

Randy was literally becoming unable to function. She described how in a grocery store or supermarket, she would suddenly experience severe anxiety, dizziness, a pounding heart, and waves of nausea as she walked up and down the aisles. Cans, cartons, and even people would merge crazily, spinning and blurring into space. It was like a nightmare. If shopping alone, she would race out of the store.

Eidetic pertains to the faculty of clearly visualizing objects and events that one has actually seen, heard, or thought up.

Soon, Randy became fearful of driving her car, especially when she was alone. Other fears appeared and mushroomed—fears of heights, escalators, water, and trains. As a child, she had suffered from motion sickness; suddenly that reappeared.

In the course of her psychoanalysis I learned that, as a child, Randy had been a slow learner and unable to read until the fourth grade, and had therefore felt stupid and inept. After high school she attended college because her mother had pushed her to do so, but she had been a mediocre student. It was in graduate school that she bloomed academically, achieving a 4.0 average. She was a late, late bloomer.

Randy confided to me that she really understood math for the first time only when she began to teach her first-grade class. She also realized that her desire to teach children mirrored her own desire to be taught how to read, write, spell, and do math.

Randy's anxieties and phobias were eventually discovered to be caused by a fascinating array and interplay of physical and emotional forces. Her agoraphobia* was due in part to her fear of becoming dizzy and losing her balance with nothing or no one to hold on to, and partly to her inward desire to leave a husband she did not love. Her other phobias were found to be caused by inner-ear mechanisms required to process motion and visual-related sensory signals. Her inner-ear–related dyslexic symptoms caused her to feel dumb and inept despite her academic degrees.

In a sense, even Randy's marriage was determined by her dyslexic disorder and the resulting emotional scarring. She had married a man she did not love simply because he felt her to be smart and tolerated her "crazy" and "stupid" fears.

*Agoraphobia is a fear of walking across large, open spaces.

3
A Simple
but Comprehensive
Concept of Dyslexia
and Its Treatments

I WILL NOW SKETCH A COMMONSENSE—AND PROVEN—CONcept of the mechanisms characterizing and defining dyslexia. This concept will easily and naturally account for all the symptoms voiced by my patients, past and present. Moreover it will prove immeasurably helpful in accounting for all the symptomatic improvements resulting from medications as well as other therapies. By carefully reading the various mental, educational, emotional, behavioral, and physical characteristics responding to medication (Chapter IV), you will see and understand the many different mechanisms responsible for and determining the complex, multidimensional disorder called dyslexia.

This conceptual sketch of dyslexia is the latest that I developed, and is the one I currently use successfully with my patients. I hope you, too, will benefit from it.

Dyslexia, as defined by the various symptoms highlighted in this book, is due to an inner-ear dysfunction. Simply stated, the inner ear serves several crucial functions, including these four:

(1) It acts as a guided-missile computer system—guiding our eyes, hands, feet, and various mental and physical functions in time and space. Thus, a disorder within this system may deflect our eyes while they reflexively and automatically fixate and sequentially track letters, words, and sentences while we read. The dyslexic's reading process is characterized by letter, word, and sentence fixation and tracking difficulties, requiring compensatory slow read-

22

ing, fingerpointing, the use of cards, etc. What's more, the resulting visual scrambling will trigger the insertion and omission of words, the illusion of new words formed from word parts separated by unseen distances, etc. Frequently words will be experienced as blurred or in movement, requiring compensatory blinking and squinting in order to restabilize the drifting input.

Inasmuch as the tracking is coarse and jerky, the reading process becomes tiring and unpleasant. Often these dyscoordinated or clumsy eye movements, mistakenly referred to as apractic, keep retargeting the same words in a sentence over and over again, a process clinically labeled ocular perseveration.

If the hand holding a pen is misguided in space, our writing will look "discombobulated" or "dysgraphic." Most often the writing will drift off the horizontal if unlined paper is used and if concentration and effort are not used to extraordinary degrees.

If our hands, our feet, or our speech mechanisms are not accurately guided in space and time, a wide range of dyscoordinated, clumsy acts or "Freudian slips" will occur ("dyslexic slips").

(2) The inner-ear system also acts like the vertical and horizontal knobs on a television set. It fine-tunes all motor (voluntary and involuntary) responses leaving the brain and all sensory responses coming into the brain.

If voluntary motor responses leaving the brain are improperly fine-tuned, one's motor acts become dyscoordinated and imbalanced, resulting in delayed speech; impaired ability to walk; difficulty tying shoelaces, buttoning buttons, zippering zippers, holding and using writing implements; and speech disturbances, i.e., slurring, stuttering, etc.

If involuntary motor responses leaving the brain are improperly fine-tuned, then toilet-training delays may arise, as well as such symptoms as bed-wetting and soiling.

If the sensory input to the brain is improperly fine-tuned, then this input will drift or scramble. The thinking brain, however bright, receiving drifting, scrambled input will have difficulty with interpretation, memory, and concentration. If the drift is 180 degrees, then reversals occur, both for incoming and outgoing signals.

Even a genius watching and/or listening to a drifting input (or a drifting TV channel) will have great difficulty remembering and concentrating on the picture seen and heard. Variations in the drifting will account for variations in the degree of clarity. Some segments will be seen and heard clearly, while others will only partially be seen and heard, and others will be completely blurred out, resulting in compensatory guessing and even illusions.

If this very same genius is asked about the content of what he observed on the TV show, he will not be able to answer too many questions. And if this genius is unaware that his difficulties are due to the TV image's drifting, then he will instinctively feel stupid, regardless of his IQ. In fact, the smarter he is, the more frustrated he will become and the dumber he will feel.

Most of the time, compliments make bright dyslexic kids feel worse. These kids know they are not able to grasp, remember, and reproduce information as well as their classmates or as well as their instincts and feelings tell them that they should. Reassuring these children that they are smart when they instinctively feel frustrated and stupid often makes them feel worse. They feel they are being lied to in order to make them feel better, to make them feel less stupid. Thus they conclude that they really *are* dumb; otherwise the compliments and reassurances would not be necessary.

In other words, bright dyslexics are instinctively aware of the many difficulties they have, and therefore react with feelings of stupidity. *Although reassurance does not reverse feeling stupid—and in fact, may seem to heighten it—it is nevertheless crucial because it keeps dyslexics going and striving until compensation occurs—if it occurs.*

Criticism, on the other hand, is felt very deeply, for it reinforces their gut feelings of stupidity, resulting in a deeper sense of inadequacy.

How can a teacher help but view these children as "stupid," "indifferent," and "defiant," especially if the teacher is viewing them as if from the backside of the TV set? If, by analogy, the teacher does not see the drift, he will naturally assume that the child is watching a simple, clear TV picture. Thus, he cannot comprehend the resulting errors and learning disabilities. Moreover, the child watching the drifting TV channel will lose his concentration and become distracted and restless. He'll want to get away from this frustrating input and shift TV channels.

By analogy this experience is very similar to how one reacts to motion sickness. Instinctively one wants to eliminate the input, either by fight or flight.

If a child can't play hooky or change his channel in school by means of distracting mechanisms, he'll fight. If his anger and fight are inwardly directed, he'll become depressed and give up. If his anger is acted out, he'll be viewed as a behavior problem with disruptive tendencies. Children will sometimes unconsciously behave in a manner that provokes authorities to suspend or expel them from school, thus attempting to get out of a most frustrating and humiliating situation. At other times, underlying guilt associated with feeling stupid and inadequate will trigger mechanisms that invite punishment and consequently alleviate guilt—a most unfortunate cycle. If, on the other hand, a child tries to avoid the frustrating drifting channel altogether, he'll be labeled as a "school phobic."

In order to understand all the variations and complexities of the dyslexic disorder, one has to carry the TV analogy a few steps further.

Picture the brain as a giant TV set with millions and millions of specific channels. Imagine each separate event as being independently processed on its own wavelength or TV channel. Thus, one channel may drift while another remains fine-tuned. One channel may drift mildly while another is completely blurred out. One channel may drift vertically while another drifts horizontally.

One channel may drift from right to left while another drifts from left to right. On and on the possibilities go, accounting for the diverse combinations of symptoms seen from patient to patient and from sample to sample.

Furthermore, the fine-tuners may vary in function from moment to moment, depending on a series of known and unknown variables and circumstances. Spontaneous variations in the fine-tuning mechanisms may result in corresponding variations in symptoms from time to time, most often beyond the individual's control. Allergies or seasons or foods may trigger signal drifting, accounting for regression in spring and fall or when sugars and dyes are present in the diet.

(3) The inner ear is also a compass system. It reflexively tells us spatial relationships such as right and left, up and down, and front and back. If this compass system isn't working efficiently, one must use one's brain to devise such consciously directed compensatory methods as wearing a ring or a watch on one hand, or recalling which hand has a scar or was broken or was used to pledge allegiance.

This compass system directs all body functions: sensory, motor, speech, thought, even biophysical patterns. Moreover, one sequence may be misdirected or scrambled while another remains unaffected or compensated for and is seemingly unaffected.

(4) The inner ear also acts as a timing mechanism, setting rhythms to motor tasks. A disturbance within this system may result in difficulty in learning to tell time and sensing time. Frequently, dyslexic children do not know *before* from *after* and can't sense whether a minute, an hour, or several hours have gone by. Accordingly, dyslexic individuals may become "compulsively" late or early. Speech timing may be off, resulting in slow or rapid talkers and even dysrhythmic talkers, or stutterers.

Any combination of these inner-ear mechanisms may be impaired. Similarly, any mechanism may be compensated for, or even overcompensated for. By recognizing that the impaired mechanisms underlying dyslexic symptoms are in a dynamic equilibrium with compensatory factors, a concept of symptom formation evolves in which each symptom is viewed as a result of opposing forces, dysfunctioning and compensatory. If gifted functions are also taken into consideration, as are self-corrective versus regressive forces, then we have truly arrived at the concepts needed to understand dyslexics and their fascinating disorder.

The above-described inner-ear mechanisms and concepts have resulted in the first comprehensive explanation of *why* and *how* the various theories about dyslexia and their corresponding therapies, including my own, work or do not work.

In discovering that dyslexia is due to a dysfunction of the inner-ear system, and realizing that anti–motion-sickness medications helped strengthen the inner ear's capacity to handle motion input and balance/coordination output (thus alleviating the various sensorimotor symptoms characterizing motion sickness), I reasoned that these very same medications may indeed improve the ability of the inner-ear system to fine-tune and process the *total* sensory input as it does the motion input, and the *total* motor output as it processes the balance and coordination difficulties noted in motion sickness. Indeed, this reasoning was clearly and decisively validated when dyslexics were successfully treated with a variety of anti–motion-sickness and related medications, and their favorable responses were carefully recorded. A series of typical medication responses will be presented in the following chapter and the varied sensorimotor improvements noted.

The wide range of expected and unexpected improvements due to my medical treatment more than justifies my theory of the inner-ear system as the fine-tuner for the brain's entire sensory input and motor output.

Now that you better understand why and how various medications I use help dyslexics, you must be curious about the mechanism underlying the favorable responses reported by allergists and nutritionists, occupational therapists, optometrists, psychologists and psychiatrists, chiropractors, dentists, and educators. Until now, most theories unwittingly confused and reversed hidden dyslexic causes with the resulting symptomatic effects.

An understanding of why various therapies work or do not work may significantly contribute to every professional's ultimate aim—a meaningful, multidisciplinary, and interdisciplinary cooperative approach. It is anticipated that this understanding will lead to new and better ways of helping dyslexics, regardless of the professional's title or the name of the therapy.

Inasmuch as dyslexia was found to be caused by an inner-ear disturbance, and in view of the fact that niacin, related B vitamins, and minerals were reported as sometimes improving inner-ear–related symptoms, the findings of nutritionists in dyslexia became readily understandable.

Nutritionists have published reports of improvement in dyslexic symptoms when vitamins and minerals are appropriately used. Other researchers have found that niacin, related B vitamins, and minerals may improve vertigo or dizziness resulting from certain inner-ear disorders, especially Ménière's disease. Ben F. Feingold, a noted allergist, recognized that sugars, dyes, and various other allergenic substances *may* aggravate such dyslexic symptoms as hyperactivity and distractibility. Accordingly the elimination of these substances leads to a corresponding symptomatic improvement. In my experience, allergies merely magnify or intensify dyslexic symptoms. They typically do not cause dyslexia.

Generally speaking, any harmful process or substance, whether stress-related, allergic, infectious, or toxic in nature, may impair or disrupt inner-ear functioning, aggravating a dyslexic disorder.

Occupational therapists and optometrists have reported academic as well as coordination improvements when dyslexics perform various motion-related and/or eye-training exercises. Inasmuch as the inner-ear system controls all body and eye movements as well as motion-related activities, and in view of the fact that practice leads to improvement in the specific motor task practiced, it seemed reasonable to assume that practicing motor activities could result in an improvement in the inner-ear mechanisms governing them. However, one must still account for the reported academic improvements when only motor exercises are performed. In other words, how and why will a child read, write, and concentrate better if he is given eye exercises or asked to participate in various balance and coordination tasks? The answer is not very difficult to obtain if one goes back to my previously described concept of dyslexic mechanisms and functioning.

If repetitive motor tasks indeed improve underlying inner-ear mechanisms, and if we assume that this improvement extends to, or is transferred to, neighboring inner-ear circuits or channels, then we can readily explain the generalized improvements that sometimes occur when specific "TV" circuits are strengthened by repetition, practice, or conditioning.

For example, if repetitive *e*ye-tracking techniques help fine-tune and condition its underlying "TV" circuit, or Channel e, and if this conditioned or improved effect is transferred to neighboring and interconnected circuits, i.e., channels r, w, m, c, t, etc., then *r*eading, *w*riting, *m*ath, *c*oncentration, and *t*ennis will correspondingly improve. However, in most circumstances transfer of functional improvements to neighboring circuits does not often occur, or is significantly restricted, accounting for the limitation of the above therapies.

When astronauts and other experimental subjects were readied for space and spun in various directions, an interesting observation was noted: Rotating someone repeatedly in a counterclockwise direction most often led to an improvement in their tolerance for counterclockwise rotations. However, it did not frequently lead to improvement in tolerating clockwise and other types of directional rotations. This observation clearly indicates how the body *specifically* adapts or changes in order to respond to correspondingly *specific* stimuli and conditions.

Fortunately, transfer of functional improvements to neighboring circuits does occur at least in certain contexts. In my practice I've repeatedly noted the existence of an jnitially puzzling and strange phenomenon: Dyslexic athletes often do best academically when in training, despite the short study time they have. Upon termination of their sports activities, due to either a changing season or an injury, a significant number of athletes report a corresponding decrease in their concentration, memory, and overall academic functioning.

At first glance, one might mistake this correlation as an excuse conjured up by athletes to justify their training time. However, this was not the case, for most often it was their parents who reported this fascinating but puzzling correlation. It therefore appeared that sports activities and exercises resulted in a transfer of function to neighboring underlying inner-ear circuits, which in turn resulted in an academic improvement. Cessation of practice led to a regression in underlying functioning, and the transfer of function was in turn eliminated or wiped out. The unexpected observations that physical exercises in dyslexics may result in increased mental capacity is in accord with the following adages: "Practice makes perfect" and "Sound body, sound mind."

Conditioning experiments in humans and animals follow a very similar pattern. If not continuously reinforced, conditioned functions and improvements disappear with time.

Over my long research career, I have repeatedly tried to understand and explain seemingly paradoxical data. I have learned that confusing events—or events occurring opposite to my expectations—invariably have a significant and important explanation if enough time is spent looking for this explanation. Most often the resulting solution to apparently contradictory or puzzling data provides us with general insights that would not emerge if confusing or contradictory data are denied or swept under the scientific "rug." As a result of this observation, I have disciplined myself to record and explain contradictions or criticism. When criticism is valid and constructive, surmounting it carries research a significant step forward. When criticism is destructive, it points out hidden flaws in the critic—flaws of which the critic and his audience are most often unaware, once again highlighting areas requiring additional attention and explanation.

The analysis of flaws, in oneself or in one's critics, has provided me with answers crucial to solving the riddle of dyslexia and dyslexic research.

Patients have occasionally reported to me some symptomatic improvements arising from chiropractic manipulation and/or dental corrections of their temporomandibular joint syndrome. Needless to say, these observations are as valid as any other type, and must be accounted for, rather than "criticized" away. It is well known that many a dyslexic will tilt his head, neck, and body in order to better read, write, and concentrate. The neck is an important integration point for the inner-ear circuitry. Perhaps, the chiropractic adjustment of these positions serves a similar purpose to that performed instinctively and reflexively by dyslexics from within.

Dental problems affecting the temporomandibular joint may often lead to headaches, dizziness, impaired concentration and dyslexialike functioning. To explain these symptoms, I have assumed that an inflammation of the temporomandibular joint may be transferred to the neighboring inner-ear system, thus either mimicking or aggravating dyslexic symptoms.

Educational therapy is as complex as it is crucial. Specific memory functions are characteristically impaired in dyslexia. Thus repetition of specific inputs is crucial if any improvement is to result. As stated earlier, specific channels of information invariably drift in dyslexics, leaving their victims relatively "blind" or "deaf" to certain inputs.

Thus, the task of educators is to find and utilize clear, open channels, as well as channels that drift very mildly, so that they may be used to impart crucial information. This teaching-learning process is very similar to what we do for the blind and deaf. However, in view of the fact that the majority of dyslexics are neither deaf nor blind, it is vitally important to improve the drifting channels via repetition or conditioning while simultaneously utilizing and stimulating open channels.

If a given sensory input drifts, its corresponding message to the thinking brain is received in a blurred, reversed, or scrambled fashion, rendering it difficult to remember and/or understand. Moreover, these drifting or blurred imprints are frequently wiped out or erased, as they are perceived as faulty. Repetition and conditioning frequently force an adaptation in which these drifting inputs are somehow finally "imprinted" or accepted for storage and memory retention. In other words the underlying inner-ear–related mechanisms processing sensory inputs have been triggered to compensate in a manner similar to the way repetitive motor tasks force an underlying improvement in the specific circuits that process these tasks.

Just as repetitive motor tasks lead to an improvement in the underlying controlling mechanisms, as well as a possible transfer of function to neighboring circuits, the repetition and stimulation used in teaching with a multisensory approach (visual, auditory, touch, proprioceptive) may also lead to both underlying and transferred functional improvements.

Each therapeutic approach has its own corresponding theory. I have tried to harmonize the successes and failures of all treatment techniques with those of my own, so that patients and professionals will have a choice as to which combination of therapies may best suit specific needs. I have saved the medical (neurologic *and* psychiatric) theories and treatment approaches for last.

Until very recently, psychoanalysts, psychiatrists, and related professionals believed child-rearing and emotional disturbances were responsible for the many learning, emotional, and behavioral symptoms characterizing dyslexics. Consequently a host of very specific subtheories and psychological mechanisms were formulated in order to account for each of the many dyslexic symptoms. Invariably psychotherapy was advised in an effort to cure and/or alleviate the emotional factors deemed responsible for the dyslexic symptoms.

The fact that psychotherapy often alleviates a dyslexic's symptoms does not prove that psychological factors caused the disturbance. Indeed, psychotherapy merely alleviates the stress and the secondary feelings of stupidity, frustration, and helplessness, factors that further complicate and destabilize an already impaired fine-tuning system. My research has clearly indicated that the psychological symptomatic fallout of dyslexia is caused by a physiological disturbance within the inner-ear system. In other words the surface psychological and behavioral symptoms are a reaction to a dyslexic's inability to function and compete normally.

The traditional neurological approach to dyslexia was significantly guided by the mistaken belief that the disorder was due to a dysfunction within the cerebral cortex—the thinking, speaking brain, the seat of IQ. This "cortical theory" has led its clinicians to misdiagnose dyslexics as having minimal brain damage, minimal cerebral dysfunction, static encephalopathy, or cerebral developmental delay, despite the *complete absence* of tangible neurological findings supporting a diagnosis of cerebral dysfunction. Clinicians still clinging to this outmoded point of view openly admit that they can neither diagnose this disorder properly nor treat it medically.

Following a rather stereotyped but traumatizing diagnosis of cerebral dysfunction, the neurologic treatment most frequently consists of referrals. Thus, patients are sent to any one or combination of the therapists, often in a biased, helter-skelter fashion.

Indeed, the cortex or thinking brain *is* impaired in dyslexics. However, it is *only secondarily* impaired. For example, if our thinking brain, however bright and intact, receives a drifting, blurred, scrambled, or reversed input, it cannot deal effectively or efficiently with the content it receives, regardless of how capable it is under normal circumstances. Thus, even the cortical dysfunction theory of dyslexia is consistent with my conviction that dyslexia is due to an impaired inner-ear system. The "cortical" theorists merely confused the *primary site* with the *secondary cause* of the cortical dysfunction.

In retrospect, psychiatrists and neurologists were similarly misled. They confused the secondary fallout of the dyslexic disorder with its primary underlying cause in the inner ear. Psychiatrists mistakenly assumed the presence of a primary psychological or mental dysfunction to explain the emotional and behavioral symptoms of dyslexia. And neurologists mistakenly assumed the presence of a primary cortical dysfunction to explain the presence of intellectual and speech symptoms in dyslexia. Each and every specialty unwittingly held on to its assumptions tenaciously.

Invariably, misdiagnosed patients are returned to the educators with either no helpful information or misinformation. Thus, educators have been given a near impossible task, one that requires Herculean effort, patience, and intuition. In the final analysis, educators were ultimately responsible for the education and treatment of the children and adults before them. They were forced to assume the total burden of the psychiatric, neurologic, pediatric, and ophthalmologic specialties, without the benefit of any meaningful medical understanding. They were forced to help, or attempt to help, millions and millions of dyslexics in the dark. Many accomplished wonders under the circumstances. Some were not equal to the task.

4
Responses
to Medication

MY AIM IN THIS CHAPTER IS TO EXPLAIN HOW AND WHY medications work to compensate for dyslexic symptoms. I encourage you to read through a series of progress reports containing the observations of parents, patients, and associated clinicians and educators. They detail and highlight the many varied responses of dyslexic patients and their symptoms to medication I recommend.

Responses such as these occur approximately 75 to 80 percent of the time with the treatment program currently in use. Several years ago, when fewer medications and chemical compounds were known to me, the favorable response rate was closer to 50 percent. I hope it will be closer to 100 percent several years from now.

To date, my studies clearly indicate that the yield of favorable responses to medication is completely *independent* of the severity of the dyslexic disorder. Over the last ten years I have treated many thousands of dyslexic children and adults with medications. As a result, I have come to recognize the importance of *two* crucial factors determining favorable responses:

(1) The pattern of signs and symptoms defining this disorder for any given patient
(2) The success or failure of the body's immunity system in filtering out or neutralizing the effects of medicines.

There exists a complex series of clinically determined correlations suggesting that specific patterns of dyslexic signs and symptoms will best respond to correspondingly specific combinations of medications. These correlations were initially highlighted by trial-and-error investigations. In other words, large numbers of dyslexic patients were treated first with one type of medication, then another, then yet another, and finally with combinations of medications. The results of these studies were carefully recorded and analyzed. Eventually correlations were established between patterns of dyslexic signs and symptoms and the medications to which these patterns responded most favorably. It is hoped that ongoing computer studies will help further define these therapeutic correlations, so that specific patterns of dyslexic functioning may be more predictably and therefore more efficiently treated.

There also exists a currently undefinable and unpredictable complex interaction between medicines and the specific ways the body's immunity system reacts to them. Were all currently utilized medicines "accepted" by the body's immunity system, the current response rate by dyslexics to medication would be closer to 100 percent rather than 80 percent. Unfortunately the body's defense mechanisms cannot always distinguish good from bad foreign substances and chemicals. As a result of this relatively "blind" filtering system, many potentially beneficial medicines are rejected and thus have no chance to help. On the other hand, medicines that do penetrate our defensive barriers may result in significant improvements.

Not infrequently, medications will work wonders initially. Then their therapeutic effect appears to decrease with time or when use is interrupted. It is as if the body develops a tolerance or resistance to the medications, rendering them ineffective. This observation is noted with many medications, not just the ones I use for the treatment of dyslexia. Often, changing the medication restarts the favorable response, clearly indicating the highly specific nature of the immunity system and its associated rejection and filtering mechanisms.

The specificity of the immunity and filtering mechanisms is most apparent when observing how one medication will result in a favorable response while a host of very chemically similar structures will either have no effect or result in side effects ranging from irritability, tiredness, and moodiness to an intensification of the very dyslexic symptoms for which the medication was intended.

Not all responses to treatment are black and white or all or nothing. Most often there are gradations of responses. To explain these variable responses to medications, I was forced to assume that the degree of the favorable response is significantly dependent upon the degree to which the body's chemical defenses reject or accept the medication. Total rejection results in either no response or side effects. Partial rejection results in partial improvement. Minimal or no rejection (i.e., acceptance) results in dramatic improvement.

Inasmuch as my success rate has greatly depended upon my becoming increasingly experienced with larger numbers of medications in more varied doses and combinations, it appears safe to assume that in the future there may be a 100-percent response rate. There is only one variable crucial to this prediction: Researchers must supply us with greater numbers of safe medications whose chemical structures are capable of improving the inner-ear dysfunction that has been demonstrated responsible for the dyslexic syndrome. The greater the number of medicines available, the greater the probability of finding one that will prove effective for any given patient.

What Medications Are Helpful in Treating Dyslexics?

To date, I have found a wide-ranging series of chemical structures helpful, including anti–motion-sickness medications, antihistamines, stimulants, antidepressants, and vitamins.* All these various chemical groupings were found to improve inner-ear functioning, albeit in different ways. I have come to view them all as "fine-tuners" of the inner-ear system. Moreover, each chemical structure was found to fine-tune a specific pattern of sensorimotor channels, suggesting that combinations of chemicals would result in the best possible response. Indeed, clinical studies have confirmed this prediction.

Readers are reminded that no medicine—even if it is available over the counter—should be taken without a doctor's advice. Side effects from the wrong medicine or dosage include irritability, tiredness, moodiness, and even intensification of dyslexic symptoms. Although some medications I use are sold over the counter, I advise parents not to treat children or themselves without the approval and supervision of an experienced physician. As stated earlier, all medicines, however "simple," may have

*Their specific chemical substances are listed in Appendix A.

side effects—sometimes serious—particularly when taken in improper doses or at the same time as other medications. In fact, I do not know why some of these medications are even sold over the counter, inasmuch as they affect a significant number of wide-ranging brain functions. Such medicines should be prescribed and supervised by knowledgeable physicians. Antihistamines and seasickness medications have infinitely greater potency and effects than their names may imply. Their purchase should not be taken lightly! Furthermore, potentially effective medications may intensify dyslexic symptoms if the dose is too high for any given patient. Thus, vertigo, nausea, motion sickness, headaches, balance and coordination difficulties, moodiness, phobias, and bad temper may all intensify unless therapeutic doses are carefully controlled and monitored.

How Do I Determine the Best Doses?

Contrary to what may be written in medical journals, *The Physician's Desk Reference,* and pharmaceutical books, my clinical experience in treating dyslexic children with antihistamines and seasickness medications clearly indicates that therapeutic doses are significantly independent of such factors as age and weight. Each patient has his own specific sensitivity and reactivity to medications, his own personal threshold. As a result, a sensitive adult may need only one-eighth of the recommended dose, whereas a child may benefit from twice the average dose.

Traditionally recommended doses are most often too high for half the patients and not high enough for the other half. For this reason I start all patients on approximately one-quarter of the average therapeutic dose. Their responses are observed and the medication is either lowered or increased, depending on the results.

How Do These Medications Work?

No one really knows the way or ways these medications work in treating dyslexia. The simplest and probably the most accurate explanation is based upon the analogies I have used to explain the dyslexic symptoms resulting from an inner-ear dysfunction:

• If, indeed, the vertical and horizontal fine-tuners are malfunctioning in dyslexia, and

- Inasmuch as the medications result in significant improvements in dyslexic symptoms,
- It is reasonable to assume that the medications result in improved functioning of the inner-ear "TV fine-tuners."

In other words the medications are assumed to help regulate and fine-tune the "TV knobs" so that the motor output and sensory input are better tuned, sequenced, and coordinated, leading to symptomatic improvement and eventual compensation.

I have repeatedly noted that each and every medication will result in a unique spectrum of symptomatic improvements: The various dysfunctioning "TV channels" in dyslexia will be more receptive and responsive to some chemical adjusters than others. This fascinating insight has led me to use combinations of medication in the treatment of dyslexia. By combining several different medications, one can obtain a greater degree of symptomatic improvement.

The medications used to treat reading, writing, spelling, and other symptoms in dyslexics were also found to improve the compass and timing mechanisms of the inner-ear system, thus accounting for the frequently observable improvement in direction, timing, and the ability to learn to tell time.

How Long Do Patients Have to Remain on Medication?

Most patients need to remain on medication somewhere between one and four years. Some patients require shorter periods of treatment, while others require longer periods. After one to four years of treatment, 80 percent of my successfully treated dyslexics will continue to do as well off the medication as they did on medication. In other words their medical treatment clinically continues to facilitate compensation even when medication is stopped.

To explain these observations, I have assumed that chemical readjustment of the fine-tuning inner-ear mechanisms may become relatively stable or permanent when used for long enough periods of time. These chemical stabilizers do not cure the disorder; rather, it is as though they teach the body how to compensate for the underlying disturbance.

Similar observations are noted in all phases of medicine. For example, high-blood-pressure medication may sometimes lead to a continued correction of this symptom despite discontinued use of the medication. Dysrhythmias of the heart and brain are often compensated for by using medications for relatively short periods of time. Stopping the medication does not frequently lead to recurrence of the symptoms even though a cure has not been effected.

Thus, childhood epileptics, for example, are helped by pharmaceutical treatment. We often stop treatment at a given age and point, without recurrence. Have we cured the underlying disorder or has this disorder merely been compensated for?

For a medical concept to have a ring of truth and the weight of conviction, it should correspond and be compatible with other, similar observations. My observations regarding the medical treatment of dyslexic symptoms are in perfect harmony with the responses noted when other medical disorders are similarly treated with medication.

Are There Dangerous Long-Lasting Side Effects?

To date, the medications I have used to treat dyslexia for the last ten to fifteen years have been around for many, many years. They have been used safely for other conditions without any observable or recorded irreversible side effects. Remember that the wrong dosage or treatment without a doctor's care can result in moodiness, tiredness, irritability, and even intensification of dyslexia's symptoms. Also, as I explained earlier in this chapter, longtime (uninterrupted) use often leads to immunity. If low doses are administered by a doctor, if patients are treated sensibly and carefully observed—if doses are appropriately interrupted over weekends, vacations, and summers—both short- and long-term side effects can be minimized and avoided.

What Short-Term Side Effects Are There?

The most common short-term side effects of the medications used to treat dyslexia are fatigue, irritability, moodiness, and intensification of symptoms. All these side effects are readily reversed by either reducing or discontinuing the doses. *No side effects should be tolerated.* They all indicate that the dose is too high or that the medication is inappropriate for the patient. All medications can and should be changed when side effects are noted.

What Do I Tell My Patients Before They Start Medical Treatment?

Medications may cause side effects and therefore incur risks, however small. All untreated symptoms cause damage or pain, emotional and/or physical. Unfortunately, nothing in life is without cost or risk. No patient or parent should agree to treatment before weighing the alternatives. No one should be *told* what to do. The possible advantages of treatment must be carefully considered by the patient *and* the doctor before a decision is made.

I present the facts of treatment to my patients and/or their parents. I may even tell them what I would do and have done in treating my own children. But I tell them to think things out for themselves and to do whatever they feel is correct. After all, clinicians and experts are only professionally responsible for the well-being of their patients. Parents are *totally* responsible for their children. They must be aware of the pain and consequences of "professional errors and unknowns."

Indeed, I respect patients and parents who raise questions and express different opinions. And I work with them to the extent that I can, in the manner I would like my colleagues to work with my decisions regarding my children's treatment.

Improvements Noted with Medications

For the sake of clarity and economy, only a handful of progress reports have been selected out of thousands for presentation. The criteria for selection were as follows: They had to be recent, typical, instructive, natural, and clear.

Analyze the recorded improvements carefully. These responses not only highlight the first and only medical treatment of dyslexia, they specifically *magnify* and thus *reveal* the complex nature and symptomatic array defining the essence and core of dyslexia. Needless to say, improvements do not occur unless an underlying corresponding dysfunction or symptom already exists.

All too often, patients do not even recognize that many of their difficulties, quirks, and idiosyncrasies are part and parcel of their dyslexic disorder. Many patients react to improvement with astonishment, often stating: "You know, I was so used to doing things this way, I thought it was normal."

Children have even more difficulty spontaneously revealing their symptoms than adults. They have no way of knowing what is normal and what is not, or how other children function. As a result, they may not reveal that they get dizzy and headachey when reading, that words get blurry and seem to bounce around, that they keep losing their place over and over again and have to use their finger or a marker, that their reading concentration and memory are poor, that letters and words appear to reverse. . . .

Denial of symptoms is a commonplace and universal reaction of dyslexic patients to their disorder. Dyslexics have difficulty recognizing, admitting, and thus revealing their symptoms to themselves and their clinicians. Consequently all scientific attempts at elucidating the various symptoms defining this riddle-packed disorder were most difficult and painstakingly slow. Were it not for the dramatic and rapid highlighting of dyslexic symptoms via their improvements on medications, my ability to map out and detail the symptoms defining dyslexia would still be in its infancy.

Few researchers develop an early and rapid grasp of the totality of the disorder they are investigating. Years of extensive effort are required to recognize even small parts of the unseen and unknown whole. Most often there initially exist significant degrees of unconscious bias and tunnel vision. One sees and recognizes only a few apparently disjointed bits of data at any given time. To succeed, this bias and resulting tunnel vision that limits our ability to see and hear what is obviously present must be resolved and replaced by the realities of the clinical situation.

Unfortunately bias is not easy to resolve. Often one doesn't even realize it is there. We deny its existence in a manner identical to the way patients deny their symptoms. Yet, bias actively distorts what we see, what we hear, and how we reason.

When I first began treating dyslexic patients with medications, I looked only for improvements in reading, writing, and spelling. At the time that was what I naively thought dyslexia was all about. I hadn't the foggiest idea that a whole range of dyslexic symptoms would improve as well: math, grammar, speech, direction, memory, time, balance, coordination, concentration, behavior, phobias, body image, etc.

Despite my initially naive and biased concept of dyslexia, I questioned my patients in a careful, open-minded fashion. Intuitively or by accident, I did not in any way restrict or direct their responses. In fact, I utilized a "free-association" or "free-flow" approach in which patients were merely told to tell me whatever they noticed *on* the medications and *off* the medications, good, bad, or indifferent. As a result of the carefully recorded and collected responses of large numbers of treated dyslexics, I was able to piece together a picture of the dyslexic disorder and its response to medications never before contemplated.

Read the medical responses reported by patients as I did. Draw your own conclusions. Make your own lists and charts. Hopefully your studies will both confirm and extend my own.

Criticism and Its Analysis

Before presenting these dyslexic responses to my medical treatment, I think it wise to present the reader with some negative, critical points of view.

Some critics have attempted to deny entirely the obvious results of my treatment. Others have termed the undeniable, positive responses to treatment as merely imaginary or wish-fulfilling placebo effects. In other words they felt that sugar pills would have had the same effect.

I pose the following questions to my critics:

- Why did other wish-fulfilling methods of treatment not work before? Surely these patients were desperate and had wanted help previously.
- Why did they respond to one medication and not to a series of others, independent of the color or the taste of the pill?
- Why did parents recognize academic improvements prior to seeing a doctor, when their children were taking antihistamines for colds and allergies?

Criticism is certainly easier than going to my office, speaking to my patients, observing them, and duplicating my results. To date, no critic has ever *disproved* any of my reported results. Indeed, many a skeptic has been scientifically converted once he witnessed my diagnostic-treatment results.

I have also been criticized for not performing "double-blind" studies—studies in which some patients are given placebos, such as sugar pills, and others "real" medications while both the examiner and patient remain "blind" to who gets what. There is some merit to this criticism.

However, I have thus far successfully managed to help over 75 percent of my patients improve while simultaneously sketching a portrait of dyslexia never before seen or imagined. All this was done without the help of double-blind studies. The results of my treatment are most clear and dramatic. In fact, the vast majority of reported symptomatic improvements were completely unanticipated and thus free from bias.

Had I *restricted* myself or my patients to viewing only reading scores, or writing scores, or spelling scores, as prescribed by the traditional double-blind method, I would have lost the forest for the trees. I would have inadvertently recorded only reading, writing, or spelling scores, since patients would not have been asked and encouraged to report freely *whatever* they noted in as unbiased a fashion as possible.

I have no regrets. Quite the contrary! I was forced to realize that traditional methods of research, however neatly and carefully reported and charted, often resulted in nothing more than a mass of data. Were this not true, dyslexia would not have remained scientifically scrambled and fragmented for over eighty-five years, a perplexing riddle requiring a solution.

Double-blind and placebo studies have their place in research. In fact, I truly believe these studies will be immeasurably more helpful now inasmuch as they can measure single variables in the context of a theme and an understood whole rather than in the preexisting scientific scramble.

I realize now why some critics are driven to *demand* double-blind studies: Underlying this need is no doubt a feeling of uncertainty as to the reality, objectivity, and honesty of their own observations.

Typical Responses of Dyslexic Patients to Medication

I will now present you with my dyslexic patients' responses to the medication I currently use. The careful study of these symptoms and responses will indeed reward you with a picture of the depth and scope of dyslexia, which cannot be appreciated or learned in any better way.

In the back of the book, I have summarized in Appendix D most of the collective responses reported to date. By the time this book is published, this list will already be outdated, for new, unexpected responses appear to surface with each additional sample of dyslexics treated.

Appendix D was quite small ten years ago. I hope that the use of new and varied combinations of medications will lead to the expansion of the improvements noted, as well as higher yields of additional significant treatment responses.

FRED AND MIKE CARTER

This letter was received from Catherine Carter, the mother of two dyslexic boys:

Fred was examined a year ago and received prescriptions and vitamins, which he took as instructed. His behavior, attitudes, personality, etc., *all* went very smoothly for the first time in his life. His teacher sent home a note after the first three days back at school in January: "I don't know what you are doing differently, but please keep it up!"

The improvement was dramatic and came about quickly. Fred's homework is no longer a five-hour chore; it takes only a few minutes most of the time now, because he doesn't have half of his classwork to do too! He finishes his classwork on time at school and sometimes so early that he gets his homework done there as well. The difference this has made in our household is absolutely amazing. Every morning used to be dominated by Fred's tantrums over going to school in the first place, over homework in the afternoons and evenings, until his bedtime. His teachers have nothing but praise for the progress he has made on his treatment program.

Fred's progress after taking vitamins and medication has been much more dramatic and far-reaching than anything previously done for him. He had tried the prescription drugs Cylert and Ritalin, the Feingold diet, an allergy diet, and visual training. The visual training helped a small amount, in very specific ways with coordination, but didn't carry over in a general way to all of his school and play activities or help the frustration levels. The inner-ear treatment you have given him has helped in a general manner with all types of coordination—running, hitting a baseball, catching a ball, *handwriting,* tying his shoes, etc. When I asked him if he could notice any changes in how he felt or how things were going with schoolwork, he said that the words no longer jumped around on the pages when he was trying to read—for the first time in his life that he could remember!

Fred remains on a closely monitored diet for food allergies; however, these seem to be going away to some degree. His allergist is the one who sent us to you in the first place, hoping to get some of the stress resolved so his system could settle down. Maybe this treatment has helped his system cope with allergies better; we really think so but certainly can't prove it. Chemicals in food still affect his behavior and performance drastically and have to be avoided.

Fred's optometrist performed a one-year follow-up developmental exam in August to evaluate improvement since the visual-training program's completion. The optometrist could see a big improvement.

We have tried taking Fred off the medication on weekends and holidays, with mixed results. Sometimes he will do fine and other times he will become cross and difficult until we resume administering at least some medication; the improvement shows inside of an hour.

Fred's brother, Mike, also showed great improvement:

We began the treatment [the day after Mike was examined by you] and it calmed him a great deal. . . . The new medications were tolerated very well.

No improvements in schoolwork were noted at home or at school until [he began taking] the prescription drug Marezine. . . . Improvement has not been as quick as with his brother but has been steady.

The temper tantrums about school and schoolwork, which began in the spring of 1982 after a severe illness and ear infection, have stopped. His grades have now returned to the A's that he used to get before the disaster struck. His attitude toward others and behavior have improved to the levels we had come to expect from him before his illness happened.

Mike's teachers are very pleased with the improvement he has shown in his schoolwork and handwriting. Math facts and times tables have become a lot easier to remember too. He is once again a cheerful little boy!

The eye squinting in the classroom that had his optometrist perplexed and [prompted him to lend Mike] a pair of glasses for reading and board work "to see if they helped, though his vision didn't really seem to warrant such a step" has now stopped. He is finishing his board work quickly and with fewer errors. All of the "dyslexic" errors are not gone, but the majority are. The frustration that he was showing is gone now. . . .

Mike's allergies have improved since the inner-ear treatment, as have Fred's, possibly due to the reduced stress of life. His allergist has been very pleased with the progress. . . .

Fred and Mike's father and I, their teachers, and their pediatrician are all extremely pleased with the boys' improvement.*

LAURA HAGAN

This letter from twelve-year-old Laura Hagan's mother was sent to me three months after she began taking medication:

Laura has made excellent progress in all areas!

*Readers are reminded that I changed the dosages when the original prescriptions caused adverse side effects (Author's note).

Her balance has improved tremendously. She could never ride a bike steadily before she was placed on medication. Now her riding is perfect, even with "no hands."

She complained of frequent headaches before, which she no longer has.

Previously, Laura would never read a book solely for pleasure, but now there have been quite a few times when she has actually turned the TV off to read!

Laura's concentration was poor and her attention span short. She was easily bored. Now she shows more interest in what she is doing and is doing it longer!

Her spelling is also better. No matter how much help or coaching she received in the past, she constantly failed and felt discouraged. Now she is achieving marks that range from 80 to 100 percent.

Laura's reading is tremendously better—she is reading at the appropriate seventh-grade level now, and her greatest advance is in reading comprehension.

Her memory or recall for math facts and concepts has also improved. She is finally making good strides in memorizing her multiplication tables and retaining them.

Laura shows more patience with herself and with others. No doubt this patience and interest is a result of the excellent progress she has made and is continuing to make, particularly with her reading ability and reading comprehension. . . . Thank you!

SAM BOWLES

Nine-year-old Sam Bowles's mother sent the following letter after Sam was on medication for one week. Although it is unusual for treatment to be effective this quickly, it does happen often enough to warrant this report's inclusion here.

I had to write and share our exciting news with you. Sam never, under any circumstances, read aloud.

As you recall, prior to leaving your offices in New York, you gave Sam medication. We immediately left for Kennedy Airport and were caught in a terrible traffic jam, arriving at the airport with only two minutes to spare. We flew from the cab into the airport, frantically searching for directions to our gate. Suddenly, Sam began to read the instructions written on the signs and the overhead, guiding us correctly to our plane. The full impact of what he had done—read the signs and overhead—did not hit me until we had boarded the plane and were safely on our way home.

Shocked, I looked at Sam—the sparkle in his eyes and his broad grin mirrored my own as he said: "I really did it, didn't I?"

JULIE CAROL ELLIS

Julie Ellis is fourteen years old. Her mother writes:

Julie has developed a keen interest in reading and has completed four books this past summer. In the past she could not read well, rarely completing more than one book in a summer.

She has improved in her coordination and balance. She is able to throw and hit a ball far better than previously, and she is now able to ride her bicycle and engage in other sports.

Julie reports that she doesn't feel as dizzy as she did before. Her ability to ride elevators, amusement rides, autos, trains, etc., is much improved. Julie doesn't suffer from motion sickness and phobias anymore.

Happily, her speech is better, increased vocabulary and more verbal content.

Julie is able to concentrate for longer periods of time and can deal better with frustration because it happens less and less.

She is more assertive at home, and at the same time her attitude is better. All in all, Julie shows a much more positive self-image.

T. J. LAGE AND STEVEN JUNGE

Lois Hanusa, a second-grade teacher in Emmanuel Lutheran School in Nebraska, wrote to me in August 1983:

This past school year, I taught two of your patients: T. J. Lage and Steven Junge. At school's end, May 26, I was absolutely sure the boys should be retained; but now with their improvement, I am considering promoting both of them.

During this summer, for eighteen days, for a half hour each day, I tutored the boys. They had seen you in April and I could see changes for the better in both of them.

I am very pleased with the boys' reactions to your medication treatment. Your solution to the problem of dyslexia seems so logical and "on target," although at first it seemed just too good to be true. I was somewhat skeptical, but am convinced now and very glad I had this opportunity to work with both T. J. and Steve and observe the effects of your treatment firsthand.

FRANK P. WATSON

Eight-year-old Frank Watson is a dyslexic child who showed remarkable progress after placement on medication. Frank went from being in a learning-disability program to being considered for his school's gifted program—in only five months.

Within two months after he was placed on a program of medication, Frank's LD [learning diabled] teacher reported that his concentration and attention span had improved considerably and his reading and general schoolwork reflected that improvement. Mrs. Watson happily added that "Frank is calmer, less irritable, and getting along well with most of his classmates. He realizes . . . that he is able to remember facts and sequential information (days of the week, months of the year, etc.) better since he has been on medication."

Two months later my office received the following enthusiastic letter from Mrs. Watson:

I simply must share with you the most wonderful news about our son Frank. After the end of the first grading period (third grade), Frank was awarded the Eager Beaver Award for Scholastic Achievement, and a few weeks later he was presented with the Citizenship Award—all firsts for our boy.

At the same time, Frank's LD teacher called us for permission to have him retested and reevaluated because of the great strides he had made in reading and other academic areas and behaviorally as well. I gave permission.

I was then called by the school and requested to attend a conference about this new evaluation. His LD teacher enthusiastically reported that she could see *no signs* of any learning disability! I was also asked to give my permission to have Frank tested for the gifted program. I was so shocked and happy I almost fainted. I quickly signed my consent.

This does not mean that Frank will be accepted into the program, but it is quite an honor even to be considered for such a placement! The more so for Frank, who had been in the LD program for three years!

With each day, we see a happier, calmer, more well-adjusted boy developing—one who eagerly anticipates going to school to learn and to be with his friends. It isn't only Frank who has profited from seeing [you] but our entire family as well. Daily, we thank God; you, Dr. Levinson; and Frank's strong determination to do well in school.

TED AND RITA POWERS

Ted and Rita Powers are a ten- and fourteen-year-old brother and sister. This letter came to me from their father:

Watching a rerun of *Donahue!* my eyes filled with tears of joy and gratitude. (And tears come rarely to a forty-one-year-old soldier who has seen a great deal of life.) You see, it was on that show that we first saw and heard you speak. [My wife's and my whole lives] and those of our children were turned around as a result.

As I am writing this letter to you, my son Ted is playing soccer, a game that previously filled him with fear. This season he joined the team and is having the time of his life. He has also begun to play football with the boys in the neighborhood. It is such a joy to us to see him happy and having fun with boys his own age.

Ted is also doing much better academically. His problems with letter and word reversals and right/left confusion don't bother him anymore. He even does his reading and math homework without being pushed and without trying to extract the answers from his mother or me.

Our daughter Rita, who suffered from recurring nightmares and fears and anxieties, also appears to be better since medication. She is calmer and more relaxed. Throughout the summer I noticed she was reading much more than she ever had.

The new semester grades have just been announced and she told us she received a 99 percent in her accounting course and an 85 percent on an assignment having to do with business accounting terminology. I hope this is a portent of the future, because last year her overall average was a *D*.

MINDI KNOWLES

Fifteen-year-old Mindi Knowles's mother wrote the following letter one year after her visit:

All the scholastic help we provided for Mindi didn't help her one bit until you placed her on medication. We see improvement in her school work, grades, and sociability.

Mindi is able to write compositions now and receive good grades. Her ability to spell has improved tremendously. Mindi said to us one day "I sure wouldn't want to be in high school the way I was—ugh! All *F*s!" We didn't realize how handicapped she was until we saw the real child emerge from the fog, the daze of dyslexia.

Mindi is able to focus her attention and concentrate on a particular subject and is more alert to her surroundings. She is even able to deal with a very aggressive fourteen-year-old sister. Again, this is something she was not able to do successfully before.

Socially, Mindi isn't on the outside anymore. She no longer looks or acts as if she is spaced out or daydreaming. To see Mindi function as she now is is truly a joy.

I recently received a letter from Dr. Stibel of the Great Falls, Montana, Optometric Group, in which he informed me that he had examined Mindi in 1981 and found her to be lacking in the areas of eye tracking, figure-ground discrimination, short-term visual memory, and phonetic word-analysis skills. He also stated that he examined Mindi after she had been placed on medication: "[Mindi's] eye-tracking, figure-ground discrimination, and phonetic word analysis skills were all significantly improved."

JAN HATCH

Another parent wrote about her fourteen-year-old son, Jan Hatch:

> We are extemely pleased with the results of your treatment of Jan. He is particularly gifted in mathematics and computer science, and it is gratifying to know that his problems no longer stand in the way of a good education in this field. Thanks to you.
>
> Jan has shown significant improvement in several important areas:
>
> *Memory:* He remembers to write down homework assignments, to do the homework once he gets home, and to take the homework back to school.
>
> *Balance/coordination:* Jan doesn't trip or seem as clumsy as before. He received an *A* in gym, a first for him because he never performed well athletically. He even qualified to test for a black belt in a martial art. His movements in general are quicker and smoother. He doesn't move back and forth when he is speaking, something he's done since he was a small boy.
>
> *Concentration:* Jan says that he thinks more clearly now and he is able to concentrate much better.
>
> The most notable difference since medication treatment is in Jan's grades. He has gone from a *D* or *C* student, with an occasional *A* or *B*, to an *A* or *B+* student. He received five *A*'s and two *B*'s this last quarter, qualifying him for Honor Roll!
>
> Everyone has noticed the differences in Jan, and he is particularly heartened by all of this.

RONALD WEBB

This report on Ronald Webb, seventeen years old, arrived two months after he began medication:

> Ron's reading is easier, fluent, and faster, and his reading level has improved with tutoring. Although his spelling memory is not much improved, he does not reverse letters anymore.
>
> Ron has noticed a big difference in his balance and space orientation. He bike rides and skates better. In school he does not experience the occasional confusion and disorientation he was sometimes prone to. Also, he does not bump into school walls and doors as he did before. He does not fall or trip as he used to, either.
>
> All of Ron's teachers have noticed some changes. In fact, his art teacher remarked about it before she knew he was on medication.
>
> Ron is a lot happier with himself. He notices things he never did before,

such as the texture of walls and fabrics, the designs in rugs, the texture of different wood grains, etc.

His grades have always been good, but he had to work very hard to achieve them. Now it all seems easier for him. Thank you!

STEVEN BROWN

Steve, seventeen years old, exhibited marked improvement toward school and life situations in general, said his mother:

Steve's mood is also more optimistic: Two and a half years ago he painted his room a dark green color; six months ago, he painted it white. He never cared much about keeping his room neat and attractive, but now he does.

I can't help but believe that the colors reflect Steve's feelings about himself and the world around him.

Even school has become less of a tense situation for him. His untimed SAT scores showed a marked improvement of about 80 points!

We are all so pleased.

GALE MARTIN

For much of her life, Gale Martin, forty-two, was plagued with hyper-activity as well as fears of heights and confined places. She also manifested a host of dyslexic symptoms related to reading, writing, attention span, and concentration. When she was placed on medication, she wrote that she experienced significant improvements:

I can now paint in my studio for long periods of time, something I had been unable to do before.

I am much better about heights and confined places; they don't seem to bother me as much as they did.

My writing, reading, concentration, and memory seem better too.

JOHN FRANK

John, six and a half years old, was referred to me because of academic difficulties. He had the third highest IQ for his grade, the 96th percentile nationally for second graders. According to teachers, he was an "under-achiever."

John's difficulties were:

• Reading on a lower grade level than his comprehension ability indicated

- Memory instability for letters and words
- Letter and word reversals in reading and writing
- Tracking problems that were responsible for his slow reading
- Poor handwriting—angulation and reversals.

On medication John has shown steadily increasing progress in the following areas:

- Basic reading skills
- Reading and math skills (he is now on grade level); displayed marked handwriting improvement
- Concentration and attention span, as verified by his parents and his violin teacher.

A detailed report outlining John's difficulties and the basis for the difficulties—dyslexia—as well as recommendations for the teachers was mailed to his school. However, the report was ignored and John continued to be termed an underachiever or a victim of "maturation lag." It almost appeared as if the child were being punished for having a high IQ while simultaneously experiencing academic problems in school.

John's parents, both professionals, arranged to meet with the principal of the school, a reading specialist, the school psychologist, and his teacher. They brought a copy of my medical text *A Solution to the Riddle Dyslexia* to the conference. Mrs. Frank wrote to me regarding this meeting:

> The faculty had seen copies of your book review outlining the main concepts of the book. They came to the conference and admitted that they couldn't understand the book review, let alone the book. We explained the book, at their request; they were attentive, but at the end of the conference they all agreed that our son's problem was a maturational one, not dyslexia.
>
> Our son is the only child in our town to have dyslexia, according to our school officials, but right across the river, in the next town, the school district has special classes for dyslexics.

Obviously, all school systems are not characterized by such stereotyped, biased thinking, and many reflect a more objective, rational approach, appreciating the importance of receptivity to new scientific and clinical theories to promote the physical, emotional, and educational welfare of our young people.

DAVID GREENFIELD

David Greenfield's parents wrote the following about their thirteen-year-old son:

Within the two-month period that David began taking his medication, his reading level improved from grade 4.5 to 7.1 and the intelligence tests given to him by the school psychologist indicated that he qualified for placement in a program for mentally gifted children.

In other areas, we see a marked change in David's behavior. He is calmer and less hyperactive. His frustration tolerance has improved, but he still flies off the handle from time to time. His concentration, memory, and auditory perception have also improved greatly. In school he is well liked by most of his teachers, but he still has retained some of his overtalkativeness, which tends to annoy some others.

David has not received any grade lower than a 94 percent on any paper he has done this year. He is doing especially well in math, social studies, and, believe it or not, English. He is also enjoying art, music, and sewing. Also, he has completed a very successful year in religious studies and Hebrew. Since he had never been able to learn any Hebrew before, he had to start from the beginning, but he has caught up satisfactorily with his classmates.

Recently, David's application to the William Penn Charter School was accepted. (This is the oldest private school in the country and maintains extremely high standards.) David's sense of accomplishment and self-confidence has been greatly boosted. He feels a lot better about himself, and he has quite a bit of insight into his own behavior.

None of this could have happened without your treatment. David takes his medication regularly, none on the weekends. Sometimes he misses the evening dose, and we can both tell the difference on those days! See you on our revisit.

MARK YILMAZ AND SCOTT ROTHSTEIN

This report is from the director of the Long Island School for the Gifted and concerns two students: Mark Yilmaz, six years old, and Scott Rothstein, nine:

Mark couldn't sit still long enough to learn anything and he could not learn to read. His intelligence revealed itself in his ability to solve mathematical problems. When math concepts were introduced to him orally, he was able to complete tasks in this area comparable to an eight-year-old.

Although his mother tried all programs suggested for dyslexic children, his reading ability did not improve and his visual skills and auditory integration continued to be weak.

After Mark saw Dr. Levinson in 1982 and was placed on medication, the results were remarkable. In spring 1983, when he was given standardized reading and math tests, his scores placed him in the highest percentiles.

Scott has an IQ of 180. He was a hyperactive child who kept everyone on the go.

He learned very quickly and was at least four grade levels above the norm in all disciplines, but he couldn't express himself on paper. He was also very disorganized. There was some attempt to give him help via the learning disability specialist. . . . Little was accomplished through this method.

In March 1983, Scott was taken to Dr. Levinson. He was placed on medication and vitamins. His behavior improved dramatically and we are working on his writing problem.

CHRIS JOHNSTON

Chris Johnston is twelve years old and in fifth grade. His mother wrote:

Your book finally reached Boise! Thank you for writing *A Solution to the Riddle Dyslexia* and enabling us to understand our son's reading problem.

He was diagnosed in the second grade as having a reading problem by the University Reading Center in Boise, but Chris was never diagnosed as dyslexic. He was in a special reading class for four years and is presently in Reading Disabilities, in connection with the fifth grade.

After reading your book, I became convinced Chris was dyslexic.

After he was placed on medication, we noticed immediate improvement in his reading and writing skills, in his balance and coordination, and in his ability to deal with frustration. His teachers noticed too.

After a year on medication, Chris is like a new child! His math is on grade level and his reading has gone up a whole grade level!

Words can not say enough to thank you for helping us by ending our years of frustration.

ESTHER PORTER

Esther Porter's parents report on their eighteen-year-old daughter:

Esther's improvement is just fantastic—almost a miracle to us. Her grades are now *A*'s and *B*'s and she will graduate from high school one semester early.

She is continually reading and writing, now that she has experienced this success. She is even talking about becoming a writer and has written a few short stories and plays. She seems able to communicate her thoughts so much better—verbally and in written form. This her tutor has told us, confirming our own observations.

Also, Esther's psychologist sees improvements in her behavior. She is calmer and her rashes are clearing up; the night activity that upset her no longer does. If you recall, she felt as though the stars in the sky and high bridges were falling as she looked at them in the evening. And most wonderful—she is finally coming out of her shell. Esther got herself a job, selling three hours a day in a department store. We are finally succeeding!

CHERIE OTTO

A patient named Cherie Otto, twenty-three years old, wrote the following report:

> My spelling and writing have improved, primarily because I can pick out my own mistakes. I never was able to do that before.
>
> My balance and coordination, eye coordination, and memory for things in a series have also improved. I am able to remember multi-stepped commands or instructions because my auditory retention is much improved.
>
> I find I can concentate better and my attention span is longer. Therefore, my organizational skills are better and I have more patience with myself. I don't lose things as frequently as I did.
>
> If for some reason I forget to take my medication, my close friends remind me. They can tell from my behavior.
>
> I finally passed my chemistry test after five failures!
>
> Both my schoolwork and my personal life have improved greatly since last year.

KIMBERLY PRICE

Kimberly Price's mother wrote about her eight-year-old:

> I have been very happy and impressed with Kimberly's improvement on medication. I don't think I can ever express my gratitude to you for the help that you have given to my daughter. The following are the changes that we have noticed:
>
> *Handwriting:* Kimberly's writing has improved dramatically. The letters have gone from a large scrawling to being better formed and of uniform size. There are also fewer letter reversals.
>
> *Math:* She is experiencing less difficulty in math computation and appears to be grasping concepts with more ease. Her number formations are also better.
>
> *Fine motor skills:* Kimberly is doing [jigsaw] puzzles for the first time in her life. She is now able to construct puzzles of 60 to 100 pieces with relative ease.
>
> *Balance and coordination:* She is now walking in a totally upright position. She no longer needs to walk slightly bent forward in order to maintain her balance.

TODD A. BRAKE

Todd Brake's parents report the following:

We have seen a number of dramatic improvements in Todd's overall ability to perform during the year he has been on medication. We have seen progress in his comprehension of math/arithmetic, very significant improvement in his verbal skills, and development of a better attitude and high morale.

Todd was transferred from a small private school to a public high school, and he has made the transition quite well, enjoying rather than fearing the new challenges. He is doing particularly well in sports, especially with wrestling. His eye-hand coordination has improved, but tennis is somewhat difficult for him, although he is practicing hard.

5

"Trust Me, Sunshine, I'll Find You Help!"

SOMETIMES THE HARDEST PART IS LEARNING THAT THE problem has a name, and finding a professional who knows it. This mother's ordeal is typical of the frustration involved with dyslexic children. . . . "Jennifer never liked to go to sleep at night, especially without a light of some kind. One evening when she was particularly concerned about going to sleep, she asked if she could sleep with me. She said she hated to sleep all by herself. I told her that as a single parent, I had to sleep alone too. I said, 'You have your teddy bear and all these stuffed animals to sleep with you.' Her teddy bear had been a friend of long standing, and a good one at that! She finally consented to go to sleep. Later that evening, when I went up to bed, I found her teddy bear on the pillow of my bed.

"The sight of the bear on my pillow brought tears to my eyes again. Just three hours earlier Jennifer, the sunshine of my life, and I had reached a new level of frustration and anxiety.

"I had known Jennifer had a problem since she was seven months old. Most children sit up and play at that age. Jennifer sat up and fell over on her side. Some forty-four sleepless nights and four pediatricians later, we discovered severe ear infections. (Even though I had suspected such, the first three pediatricians insisted she was teething.) In a matter of days, with the proper medication and care, she was well. But her ears had been scarred to the point where they now look as though they had had draining tubes in them.

"To help her overcome her lack of coordination, I enrolled Jennifer in a ballet class when she was three. Several months later I discovered she still didn't know her right from her left. By putting a round blue sticker on her left ballet shoe, she learned to determine the difference most of the time. Her coordination and balance were not good, however, and her ability to follow a sequence of directions was poor. Jennifer also needed an outlet for a great deal of hostility. As a result, I enrolled her in a karate class when she was five. She enjoyed karate, and it has provided opportunities for her to experience a number of successes.

"Starting school was exciting for Jennifer, and she looked forward to each day throughout kindergarten. She worked well in groups and learned a great deal. Of course, there were days when she forgot her sweater or coat or lunch box or book bag, but in general she did well and loved school. (She and her friends even 'played' school.) Therefore, her first formal academic experience was a positive one.

"Jennifer frequently complained of stomachaches and headaches that seemed to be nonexistent. She had nightmares often. It was difficult to bring her out of the dream and back to reality. I had no answers and neither did her doctors.

"About halfway through the first grade, more serious problems started. At that point she was learning to read and write. She would finish some assignments but not others. There were some that she didn't even attempt. Her teacher and I were puzzled. We made games out of learning; that proved successful on several occasions, and the learning-resource teachers worked on various ideas. Some helped for a little while; others didn't work at all.

"Learning to read was difficult because Jennifer had to reread passages constantly in order to comprehend them.

"Second grade started out the same way that first grade had ended: Jennifer finished some projects and not others, and a number of assignments were never started. She seemed to lack the ability to concentrate when reading, although she could concentrate if a subject interested her. I requested that the school test her, and she tested quite well. Jennifer was not distractible in a one-on-one situation; she finished everything she was asked to do. It took some time but she did finish. She was judged to be more than one year beyond her grade level in reading and mathematics. Hence the school system suggested only psychological help. We made an appointment and spent an afternoon with a group of psychologists. They recommended that she *not* work with them; there was no evidence of any need for counseling.

"Even though she continued to have the same problems in school, Jennifer finished second grade and went on to the third. She still used her finger to point when reading or writing and had trouble remembering words she had studied an hour earlier. She had difficulty with basic math facts, such as adding and subtracting simple numbers. I bought games designed to help with mathematics, including flash cards and a math kit that consisted of plastic blocks. We worked through that kit—three times. I learned a lot of mathematics; Jennifer did too. But the next day her knowledge was gone.

"When Jennifer entered the fourth grade, she encountered the same problems. Her teachers were concerned and very helpful in that they understood what I faced each evening; in turn, I knew what they had to contend with daily. At least I had Jennifer by herself. Had I to cope with another twenty-seven students in the same room, I'm sure I would have been a wreck.

"Fourth grade brought further insight, as the multiplication tables are taught that year. What a fiasco that was! We would go over and over the multiplication tables, but she would remember only some of them. She worked very hard, because she wanted to do well, but without success. One night we *sang* them together and laughed. (She had a terrific, totally uninhibited laugh.) But I sang too fast for her. She would tell me it was all right, that she was just dumb. I tried to convince her she was not dumb, that she was indeed a very smart little lady. I could hear her cry herself to sleep that night.

"Jennifer was described by some as hyperactive. We tried the Feingold diet, which prohibits preservatives and artificial ingredients, but the diet made no difference in her progress at school or her behavior.

"Jennifer still complained of headaches. She also mentioned problems reading the chalkboard, so I took her to an optometrist. She got glasses, but the same behavior and learning problems persisted. The glasses only proved to be something else to lose.

"Jennifer's handwriting was extremely messy and the letters crudely formed. I noticed letters that were backward, mirrored. She had brought home instructions that she should practice her handwriting, so practice she did, but to no avail. I began to notice that she would capitalize words in mid-sentence. When I asked her about that, she had no answer.

"Having taught for nearly fourteen years, I felt I should know the solution to my daughter's problem. After all, there I was, with two degrees in education and nearly half the course work for a doctorate. Yet, I was unfamiliar with these kinds of problems or what to do about them. I had taught special-education classes, but I felt helpless.

"I started reading everything I could get my hands on and consulted a medical dictionary often. I realized that Jennifer had all the symptoms—not just some but *all* the symptoms—of dyslexia. I called the school and requested that she be tested again, specifically for dyslexia.

"Two weeks later I was told that my daughter's IQ was above average. Her work, they said, *when she did it,* was all above average. Therefore there was no problem. But I knew there *was* a problem. If they would just listen . . . !

"I was beside myself. The same problem that had first surfaced in first grade continued. Why couldn't we get any help? I began to search for help outside the school.

"We went to audiologists, optometrists, and pediatricians. We visited medical school teams (who are teaching *tomorrow's* doctors!). Most of them tested her. All of their cash registers jingled. None of them helped. Audiologists and optometrists suggested we see ear, nose, and throat specialists. We saw them all; *no one had the answers.* Not only was I filled with frustration, I was throwing away good money after bad. No one helped. I sobbed uncontrollably for hours.

"My patience had long since worn thin, as had Jennifer's. Her problems made her feel like a failure. I've always felt that the best thing parents can do for their child is to give him or her a positive self-image. I was a practicing positive parent; I still am. But my child had the poorest self-image! Because Jennifer sings well, I enrolled her in voice lessons so she could experience positive feelings about herself. Although she did quite well, her negative self-image remained unchanged.

"Jennifer continued to spend three hours doing homework that should have taken fifteen minutes. We argued; we got frustrated. We both lost our patience. We would end up sobbing. We would hug each other and apologize for 'losing it.' I could see that she was trying so hard. Helping Jennifer do her homework was like being a referee for an elementary-school basketball game: If you call all the fouls, you have nothing but foul shots and the kids don't learn to play the game. If I called all the fouls with Jennifer, we had absolutely no positive time together. I refused to do that.

"The school situation continued to get worse. Jennifer not only refused to turn in her homework (she was afraid it was not right, even though I checked it every night); also she did not do her classwork. She would get frustrated and throw a temper tantrum. She would make ugly remarks to her classmates and her teachers. I would get phone calls from the teacher, who told me Jennifer wasn't developing meaningful relationships with other children, that Jennifer was bossy and childish.

"I knew my daughter was crying out for help. I just didn't know *how* to help. I began to call doctors again. This time I decided they had to prove to me over the phone that they knew what I meant when I said, 'Jennifer doesn't receive and process information like the rest of us.' Some of them wouldn't talk to me unless I came in for an appointment; others indicated that they didn't know what I meant. One of the doctors who seemed to understand was an ear, nose, and throat specialist. He even knew that the condition has been likened to motion sickness and was being treated with motion-sickness medication and antihistamines. I was elated. We made an appointment.

"The doctor's first comment was 'How long ago did you first notice a hearing loss?'

"I told him, 'Jennifer doesn't have a hearing loss; in fact, she hears better than most.'

" 'We'll see,' he said, patronizingly. He brought in an audiologist, who led Jennifer away for testing. Ten minutes later, they returned. The audiologist gave the doctor a form that had been dutifully filled out. The doctor said, "This child doesn't have a hearing problem; in fact, she hears better than most!" I thought for a moment there was an echo in his office.

"He continued to examine Jennifer. He blew air into her ears. He looked inside her ears. 'Let's face it, Mrs. Scharle,' he said to me, 'maybe she just doesn't like it.'

" 'Like what?' I said.

" 'School,' he replied.

" 'Are you telling me a child who doesn't like school comes home and plays school?' I asked him.

" 'Perhaps you should see a psychologist,' he said.

"I thanked him and took Jennifer's folder to the front desk. After writing a check, we left. I was appalled. This man had convinced me he knew what he was talking about! How could I have been so dumb? Another $89 down the drain. (Outpatient testing is rarely covered by group health insurance.) What were we going to do?

"Everyone referred us to someone else. I watched Jennifer become more and more frustrated and hostile. She saw me subtract more and more from my checkbook. Family and friends recommended one counseling service after another. (It seems that a child whose parents are divorced is supposed to be emotionally imbalanced and a behavior problem. I knew better. I knew that Jennifer was a warm, loving, sensitive child with a learning problem and no self-image to speak of. She just didn't receive and process information like the rest of us.)

"Jennifer became convinced that no one understood. She spent hours trying to help me, trying to make my life easier. By folding clothes and vacuuming, setting the table and clearing it, feeding the dog and letting him out, she sought my approval because she believed she couldn't get it otherwise. She felt like a failure.

"I continued to work with her on homework assignments, but we both frequently lost our patience. I couldn't come up with a successful learning approach. Nothing we tried worked. We cried, hugged each other, rocked each other, and patted each other's back. 'We'll find an answer,' I told her. 'Your mother will find a way to help you if it kills her.' She insisted she was just dumb.

"In despair I tried to scare Jennifer into working better, a conditioning technique I had read about. I told her perhaps I was in the way. I was going to let her be responsible for her own homework. She was on her own. Remember, I said, if you are in the fourth grade again next year, the kids will be teasing *you,* not *me,* at the bus stop. And I left her to do her homework. She worked and cried and worked and cried. It still took her three hours to do fifteen minutes of work.

"Jennifer developed frustration problems at school: One day her frustration exceeded even her norm.

"Jennifer had been assigned to do a work sheet. She couldn't do it, or so she thought. When her teacher questioned her, her frustration reached its peak and she threw her notebook against the wall. Just then the school secretary called over the intercom that Jennifer's father was there to pick her up, which he did every Tuesday and Thursday. Her teacher asked another teacher to keep an eye on her class and went out to speak with Jennifer's father.

"While she was telling him that she had taken as much as she could from Jennifer, Jennifer became convinced that the other teacher (someone she didn't know) was not going to allow her to go to her father. When Jennifer insisted that the lady let her go, and the other teacher insisted that Jennifer was to stay there where she was, Jennifer got frustrated again and threw her lunch box against the wall.

"By the time I was informed of the situation, Jennifer's father had had enough too.

"What could I say? He didn't spend every evening doing fifteen minutes' worth of homework for three hours. He didn't see the daily frustration she experienced.

"Jennifer's father may have known how difficult it was for her to tell time; he may have known that she had a special system for remembering the days of the week. But he didn't know that she had a list in her book bag that said, 'book bag, lunch box, sweater or coat, homework books, assignment pad, and *you!*' (Not only had she forgotten one or more of these items many, many times, but once she caught the wrong bus and didn't come home!) Sometimes she even forgot to check the list.

"Jennifer got in my car and started crying. She was expecting a reprimand from me, a reinforcement of her negative self-image. She sobbed—as I did—all the way home. 'Why do I have to be different? Why can't I just be like everyone else?' she asked. I cried harder. My poor little girl—no one understood. The whole situation tore at my heart. We went inside and sat down. I promised her once again, 'I'll find you help. Trust me, Sunshine, I'll find a way to help you.'

"I had no idea how I was going to accomplish that miracle. I couldn't eat; sleep didn't come easily.

"One day a friend of mine noted my mood, and asked if he could help. I told him how I wished he could and gave a brief description of the problem. Surprisingly he proceeded to tell me how he had been illiterate when he graduated from high school. I listened in disbelief. The man owned his own company and was doing extremely well. Beyond that, he had graduated from college with second- and third-grade reading and writing skills. No public school system had ever helped him. It was not until he was twenty-eight and wanted to learn something on his own that a tutor pointed out what his problem was and whom he should see about it.

"My response was frantic: *'Who?'*

"He gave me the doctor's name and phone number. I had a million questions. Did it work? What did he do? How did the doctor help him? What kind of doctor was he?

"The doctor was a local optometrist. After extensive testing he had given my friend eye exercises that had to be done regularly for some six months. Yes, it had worked. He might have the answer for Jennifer; then again, he might not. It was worth a try, surely.

"First thing Monday morning I called and made an appointment. I sent my chronicle of Jennifer's development and samples of her handwriting, plus a multitude of other reports, before we arrived at his office.

"The nurse came into the waiting room and asked if I would see the doctor alone for a few minutes. Jennifer agreed to wait in the lobby. And then the warmest voice said, 'I feel like I already know you.' Somehow I knew Dr. Howard Kahn would help.

"He was pleased with the paperwork I had sent ahead. He had read it with 'incredible interest,' he said, and realized the frustration Jennifer and I had been through. I couldn't help but believe that this man would provide the assistance we needed.

"He called Jennifer in and tested her eyes. (A young boy down the street had destroyed her glasses two days earlier, so the eye test came first. This is not his normal procedure.) The rest of the tests would follow.

"I stayed in the room while he tested Jennifer and I noticed that his bookshelves were loaded with books about learning disabilities. I would have killed to get my hands on that literature just one week before!

"The eye tests provided tremendous insight into Jennifer's problem. At least some of it was due to the eyes.

"The relief I felt from having found a doctor who not only understood the problem but thought he could help is nearly impossible to describe. The knots in my stomach disappeared. My headache and furrowed brow left me on the way home. I took a deep breath and looked at Jennifer. She was singing a song with the radio. She felt the relief too.

"She now had two people to help her—her mother and her new eye doctor. She admitted to being a bit leery on the way to his office, but now it was okay. She trusted him, she said.

"I didn't tell her that the doctor had said the worst was yet to come, because I couldn't believe that myself. Not knowing what to expect was the scary thing. Jennifer and I could do anything. After all, we had made it that far.

"That night, as I kissed Jennifer good night, she hugged me a little tighter and longer than usual. 'Mom,' she said, 'you're the best mother in the whole wide world. I'm really lucky I have you.'

" 'Thank you, Sunshine,' I said. 'You're the best daughter in the whole world too.'

"I wondered what would have happened if I had had no background in the field of education. I wondered what would have happened if I were a high school dropout on welfare and food stamps and with four or five kids. What do the children do under those circumstances?

"The photographer Susan Jacobs, herself the parent of a learning-disabled child, has said, 'I feel very strongly that a parent must trust himself and the desire to help his child. He must not let himself be intimidated by people who are critical of him and think because he's concerned and worried about his child, he is an "overprotective parent." . . . As a parent, you know your child better than anyone else, and you must trust your knowledge and feelings to find the best support for your child in enabling him to feel better about himself.'

"The Foundation for Children with Learning Disabilities says, 'Let no child be demeaned, nor have his wonder diminished, because of our ignorance or inactivity. Let no child be deprived of discovery, because we lack the resources to discover his problem. Let no child—ever—doubt himself or his mind because we are unsure of our commitment.'

"There are many such children. It is estimated that 25 to 30 percent of the school-age population in this country has a learning disability. It's an invisible handicap. These children have diverse sets of characteristics that affect their development and achievement. There is no physical disability or visual characteristic to guide us in distinguishing learning-disabled children.

"This is simply the story of one child's fight for the right to learn and be just like everyone else. This story is written in the hope that no other child will have to fight as Jennifer has. I hope that no other parent has to go through the same frustration of not knowing what to do.

"Now we're on our way to success. We've found an eye doctor who knows what to do. Less than a week after our first appointment with him, a directory arrived from the Foundation for Children with Learning Disabilities. It's published by Academic Therapy Publications, Novato, California, and it lists facilities and services for the learning-disabled all over the country. These people know how to test and what one should learn in order to cope with the disability.

"Early in Jennifer's fourth-grade year, I made an appointment for her with a neurologist-psychiatrist in Great Neck, New York—Dr. Harold N. Levinson. The earliest appointment we could arrange was for May 25 of the following year, but the wait was worth it. Jennifer spent some three hours being tested and interviewed and I was interviewed as well. Technologists administered some of the tests and Dr. Levinson conducted others.

"Jennifer knew that the doctor understood. As we flew back home she quietly wrote me a note that said, 'Thanks, Mom, you're the greatest.' She knew he was going to help because he understood all the problems she'd been having. Those symptoms and quirks that made her 'different,' those that she had questioned so many times, were soon going to be corrected, and she knew it.

"Jennifer started the fifth grade as she had no other in her academic history. After a month and a half she has yet to fight with homework. She has yet to go without finishing her work in school. We have not had one cross word; we have not spent one frustrating evening together, although she still has to work harder than most of the students simply to catch up on things such as basic math facts.

"In addition to taking medication, Jennifer is currently studying with a tutor who is also a diagnostician and counselor. She has spent a number of hours working with Jennifer and her assistance has proved successful. Jennifer will begin eye exercises, too, in the next few months. Dr. Levinson has prescribed vitamins, lecithin, motion-sickness medication, and an over-the-counter cold remedy.* The difference in the child is phenomenal. She is indeed the child I raised her to be.

"I'm not a scientist; I'm an educator. But first and foremost I'm a parent who loves her daughter more than words can tell. It's been a long, hard battle, but we have gotten this far and we'll go further. Sheer determination on Jennifer's part and mine has provided a great deal of insight and progress. Luck has been on our side as well.

"Above and beyond all else, I can say this: Jennifer has taught me commitment. She has taught me patience and compassion. Most important, she has taught me to love. We are closer because of this. We love more deeply because of this. No one can possibly understand without having lived through such an ordeal. Jennifer fought for me as I fought for her and her rights. You will find no greater love than that of someone who has made the commitment to fight for you. Nor will you find greater love than that of someone who puts you before herself."

*This combination was right for Jennifer. It is *not* necessarily appropriate for anyone else (Author's note).

6
Determination

THE STONES WERE DETERMINED TO SEE THEIR SON ROB SUC-
ceed despite the ignorance and defensive malice of the "experts."

Usually youngsters of preschool age eagerly anticipate the beginning
of the school year. They can't wait to learn reading, writing, spelling,
and math, to mix with other children and enthusiastic teachers. Very few
of us aren't touched by sparkling faces, shiny eyes, and small fingers
tightly clutching prized notebooks and pencil cases. How sad, though,
when the light and joy go out of a youngster's eyes, and instead of eager
anticipation of school, there is only anxiety and even dread.

Such was the case of Robert Stone.

Shortly after starting kindergarten, Jean Stone received a call from
Rob's teacher. Rob was known to be hyperactive and distractible in the
classroom. Moreover, he was unwilling or unable to follow instructions,
and the teacher suspected the presence of perceptual motor difficulties.

Despite the Stones' attempts to remedy the classroon situation, the
situation deteriorated. The school psychologist met with Rob's teacher
and parents, reviewed *all* the findings, and strongly intimated that emotional conflicts within the Stone household were no doubt responsible for
Rob's problems in school.

Strangely enough, the psychologist's findings were in stark contrast to
what the Stones and Rob's teacher thought. In fact, Rob's teacher rec-

ognized the boy's restlessness to be a hyperactive rather than an anxiety or attention-seeking symptom. In addition, she observed his clumsiness and accident proneness and called those factors to the attention of the clinical personnel. Rob had difficulty walking through a hallway with a sloped floor without tripping or bumping into walls or other children. In the classroom he frequently dropped things and would even fall from his seat periodically. Rob's teacher advised the Stones to have Rob start perceptual motor training rather than the psychotherapy advised by the school psychologist.

The Stones' and the teacher's opinion was negated by the school's clinical team. After all, the team consisted of "experts" in child development and psychoeducational techniques. What did Rob's teacher and parents really know about him? Nothing! They were condescendingly viewed as uninformed, biased onlookers.

Had Mrs. Stone not been a teacher herself for a number of years, she might have been confused and intimidated. As it was, she followed the kindergarten teacher's suggestions that Rob be tutored and trained in perceptual and motor coordination tasks during the summer in preparation for the upcoming school year. These techniques seemed to work.

Unfortunately, Rob began first grade under fairly distractible circumstances—an added handicap for him. Four first- and second-grade classes were grouped together in one large room, separated only by shelves that were three feet high. Almost immediately Rob's inattentiveness and hyperactivity escalated. He began to wander around the classroom and even hid in the coatroom, instinctively attempting to avoid sensory overloading.

Rob's teacher was unable to control him and had to drag him out of the closet. Frustrated and in despair, she spanked him several times in front of the class. Obviously that was no solution; he just could not be controlled. As a result, Rob was placed in the library with an aide as his teacher. This situation greatly disturbed his parents.

Again meetings were called. The school clinical team's evaluation had not changed too much. Rob's problems were diagnosed as emotionally based. In addition, the team decided that there must also be some kind of brain damage present. Therefore they advised that he be placed in a hospital for a week of testing, and they recommended placement in a special school for brain-damaged children.

Understandably these proposals thoroughly surprised and shook Rob's parents. They totally rejected this whole line of "reasoning." They firmly believed their son was not brain-damaged. He was bright, responsible, and sweet, and he had never exhibited at home the behavioral problems he exhibited in school. Moreover his vocabulary and verbal skills were exceptional. Obviously something was wrong, but the Stones intuitively knew that the school clinical team's solution was out in left field. After much deliberation and in despair, they decided to send Rob to live with his maternal grandparents in a nearby state. There was no alternative; they could not afford private schooling and they obviously had to get him out of the school district he was in.

Despite their anguish and guilt, Rob's move to a new school proved to be a good one initially. He learned to read and write better in the stricter, more structured and demanding environment. However, the problems did not disappear; they were just less intense and dramatic.

Although he received additional help in reading, Rob remained six months behind his peers. And although his behavior was less of a problem, he continued to be disorganized, restless, and inattentive, and still experienced coordination problems in gym. Rob's separation from his parents also created new problems. His mother worried about him continuously and couldn't tolerate the separation. Rob's maternal and paternal grandparents—good friends for many years—suddenly began to fight among themselves over his rearing and education. Guilt and recriminations ran rampant. Rob sensed he was the cause of it all.

In an attempt to resolve the escalating concerns, antagonism, and conflicts, the Stones decided to relocate to the grandparents' town. Mr. Stone would stay behind until he completed his doctorate, while Mrs. Stone would move back to her hometown, rent a house, and rejoin her son. "Although we made this decision with such care, concern, and even sacrifice for Rob's welfare, in hindsight it all seems to have been a bad move."

Rob regressed emotionally despite his concerned mother's presence. Once a sweet, lovable child, he became morose, stubborn, defiant, even hostile. One evening he was overheard saying his prayers, "Please, God, please give me a brain!" His mother was filled with indescribable sadness, frustration, and hopelessness.

Rob felt stupid because he continued to lag behind his peers in reading, even with tutoring and continued reassurance by his mother. Yet, the Stones knew their son was bright. At times he even seemed gifted. But they couldn't explain his learning and coordination difficulties. Although Rob's six-month lag in reading didn't bother the school much, it frustrated and devastated Rob and his parents. The Stones asked the school to test him for a learning disability.

Upon testing, his IQ was found to be at least 117 in spite of his concentration difficulties and restlessness. The clinical team leader, Mrs. Harris, realized Rob was easily distracted and so she decided not to remove him from his regular classroom. Had she placed him with other distractible children, his behavior no doubt would have worsened. This decision drew a sigh of relief from Rob's entire family.

Although Rob remained in his regular classroom setting and received help from a gifted and dedicated, supportive reading teacher, Mrs. Wright, he was removed from his regular gym class. The new gym class had only one other student, a child whose legs had been amputated from the knees down. As Mrs. Stone stated, "Rob could see the obvious physical disability the child had, but he must have asked himself what his disability was. He already felt stupid. He continually called himself klutzy. What else did he think was wrong with him now?"

From this point on, Jean Stone will tell her story in her own words.

"Rob was devastated at being removed from his friends; he also felt humiliated to be placed with only one other physically handicapped child.

"We all, including his friends, tried very hard to make him feel loved and wanted. We were determined to help Rob retain his sense of worth and to keep intact one very special and lovable boy.

"Rob began the new school year in the third grade, but soon there began a repetition of the past. We had to meet with the school clinical team several times. My friend and ally, Team Leader Harris, was replaced by a Mr. Smith, who accepted the recommendation of the school psychologist and Rob's teacher without evaluating things for himself. That meeting was a nightmare! The psychologist and the teacher insisted that the child was incapable of handling third-grade material and was emotionally disturbed. The only person to object to this evaluation was Mrs. Wright, his reading teacher. She voiced her opinion that 'he was one of the most intellectually curious and sweet children that she had worked with in fourteen years.'

"This meeting and the others that followed convinced me that there was a lack of compassion or caring for Rob. These people seemed to be condescending in tone and manner, hoping to intimidate and confuse me, to manipulate me to accept their conclusions. But I would not!

"I was an educator myself for many years, and familiar with the jargon of the profession—familar also with the methods. I was therefore able to deal with these people on their own level and with their own terminology. I frequently asked myself what other parents did in similar circumstances. Do they fight against the 'experts'' edicts, as we did, or do they cower and capitulate, assuming that the 'experts' know best.

"Whichever position they take, there is heartache for the child who is the object of the controversy. However, for us there was no choice. We were determined to do what was best for our son, regardless of the consequences. Time and time again, after each painful session, I wondered where the clinical team's sense of compassion lay—that quality so essential for every good educator. Certainly this school's clinical team lacked empathy. In addition, the team was very annoyed with me because I was able to question their advice. I needed to have answers that would help my son, and I was not going to be put off or intimidated by anyone.

"Fabrications about my son's academic performance were told—that he was unable to remember math facts when math was his best subject. The psychologist insisted that Rob's stomach upsets were avoidance tactics. I told them that he had always had such upsets—not only when he had classwork to do, but also after the bus ride to school and again when he came home, after gym, or after any hectic activity. The true significance of these stomach upsets was not pieced together until our visit to you, Dr. Levinson.

"Teachers sympathetic to Rob and to us were subtly and overtly told to present a united front at the meetings and to allow the clinical team leader to speak for the team as a whole. Mrs. Wright became the butt of gossip that was spread by members of the team. It was difficult to comprehend that this slander was intended to vindicate the team's position.

"Mrs. Wright informed me that Rob had the highest IQ (by 50 points) in the private-instruction class. She knew all the children in the class, and she strongly felt that Rob did not belong with them.

"I pleaded with Mr. Smith not to place my son in the class, but he refused to listen.

"At midyear, Rob was placed in a special-education, self-contained class, the PI [private instruction] class. Our little boy was devastated. In all schools these segregated classes have stigmas attached to them, and Rob felt demoralized to be placed in such a class after our long, hard battle. Our hearts ached for him.

"We did our best to comfort him and stem the flood of tears, but by the second week of placement, Rob had undergone a transformation for the worse. He cried at the drop of a hat. He was mean to his sister, to his brother, and to us, his parents. He spent most of his school day in the principal's office because of bad behavior. He brought no work home from school. In general, his behavior was obnoxious, uncontrolled, and impulsive.

"One day I received a call from the music teacher, informing me that Rob was lying on the floor, rolling around. I was horrified and decided to see for myself.

"I went to school, spoke to his teacher, and asked to see Rob's schoolwork. The only work he had produced in a two-week period was an incomplete work sheet—at kindergarten level—with black scribbling. The teacher said she could neither reach nor control him. When I looked at that page of scribbling, I almost crumbled. Two short weeks earlier he was only six months behind third-grade level! Tears, then anger, took over—searing, hot, red anger. How dare they do this to my son?

"I removed Rob from school and informed the school clinical team, especially the psychologist, that Rob would not return to school until he was reinstated in his regular third-grade class. In the meantime I would teach him myself at home.

"In spite of threats and nasty phone calls, I stood firm in my resolve to teach our son. All I had to do was look at my son's face and I knew I had done the right thing: He was happier, performing beautifully, and soon approaching grade level! After six weeks I received a phone call from the team leader: I was told that Rob could attend his regular third-grade class. However, first a meeting between us and the team members had to be held.

"In spite of the failure of the PI class, attitudes were unchanged. The school psychologist, the school system's head of psychology, and the other team members still felt that Rob needed to be in a special class. In fact, the team leader commented, 'It's a shame Rob is so bright. . . . What good is a high IQ if you can't use it?' My mother-in-law was with me and I had to restrain her at that point.

"Once again the reading teacher, Mrs. Wright—who had taught Rob the longest and who knew him better than any other teacher—was ignored and made to feel that she had nothing valid or important to contribute to the proceedings.

"We felt extremely frustrated by the narrow-minded attitudes we encountered, but we never wavered in our resolve to have Rob placed in a normal classroom setting. We were bolstered in our purpose by our intimate knowledge of our son and the dedicated, unswerving support of the reading and music teachers.

"Rob spent the last month of school in a regular class, elated to be with his friends, but under pressure with the understanding that he must perform or be returned to the commotion, confusion, and stigma of the PI class. The balance of the year went fairly well.

"The end of the school year brought us a shocker. The school team announced that Rob should not go on to the fourth grade because his behavior was inappropriate and distracting to other students. Also, since he had not done well in the school's PI class, he should be placed in another school district's special-education program.

"Despite all our efforts, the team clung stubbornly to its position, completely ignoring the fact that their insistence on placing Rob in the PI class nearly destroyed him. The team would not acknowledge its failure, adhering to the psychology report findings that stated that Rob was emotionally disturbed, with a minimal learning disability, and therefore should be placed in an open, nonstructured classroom. We, his parents, and Mrs. Wright disagreed, contending that retention in the third grade with additional help in reading was the best way to meet Rob's needs. The illogical stance of the school's clinical team's argument was apparent to everyone but the members of the team.

"They censured Rob for his distractibility and at the same time insisted that he be placed in an extremely distractible environment. The team—almost vindictively, it seemed to us—insisted that they knew better how to meet Rob's needs.

"We consulted with a friend who was involved with the state education board. He advised us to have Rob retested by another clinical team located elsewhere, independently and at our own expense. We did so.

"This new evaluation, the support of Mrs. Wright, and the illogical stance of the school team's proposal forced the district superintendent to override his team's recommendation. Rob would be retained in the third grade with a teacher who was reputed to maintain a strict, structured classroom. We were elated over this decision.

"However, in the same breath that the superintendent announced his decision to override the proposal, he peremptorily said, 'What will you do when this fails? I know your son will become a drifter throughout school and eventually a nobody. The monkey is on your back now.'

"It was at this time that we saw Dr. Levinson, on the Phil Donahue Show. For the first time my husband, our parents, and I were truly able to understand what Rob had been dealing with. No longer could we blame Rob or ourselves—no longer could we even think to ourselves that Rob was 'slow' or 'not quite right.' Not that we ever consciously verbalized these thoughts, but they nevertheless were there, and perhaps, unbeknownst to us, they were conveyed to Rob.

"Suddenly, Rob's inability to traverse certain school halls without falling, tripping, or bumping into other children became plausible in the light of his inner-ear dysfunction. Suddenly it was as though our characterization of Rob as a perfectly lovable and intelligent human being was validated.

"Most important, I could explain to Rob what he had. He quietly listened while I showed him pictures and sample writings of other dyslexics from your book. He looked into my eyes and was totally attentive.

Finally, he asked, 'Is that why I always get sick on a swing?' I never knew that that had happened. All the pieces began to fit together—the stomachaches, the sensory overloading and upset when too much was happening too fast, the inability to sit still for more than a few seconds, etc.

"I called and made an appointment with Dr. Levinson. He examined Rob and determined that he was dyslexic.

"We began to have good results almost immediately. Rob was able to negotiate the halls, doorways, and steps without holding on to the walls. After only the third day of medication the reading teacher observed that Rob was reading faster than her fingers could track the lines. Rob's spelling and punctuation also showed improvement and have continued to do so.

"When Rob wrote compositions, he used to use only words that he knew how to spell, but between memory and spelling improvement and teacher encouragement and understanding, his creativity in writing has amazed us.

"For the first time Rob has been able to attend services in the old log-cabin Protestant church to which the entire family belongs. He had never been able to attend services because the white masonry and dark cedar logs horizontally laid made him nauseous. Now Rob not only attends services but also sings in the choir. His position is in the middle of the line, on the middle step; he stands straight and does not weave, stumble, or fall—another fantastic first!

"Due to motor coordination–balance improvement, Rob was once again placed in a regular gym class. His medication, plus his tremendous drive to perform well, have produced amazing results. Within a few months of the change, he became captain of the hockey team and an effective player—truly amazing when you consider that he had been unable to run twenty feet without falling down!

"Rob experienced two other successes that were a great source of pleasure to him and that emphasized how far he had come. He entered a roller-skating race with his classmates. The race took place in a large indoor rink—and he won second place! He also competed in a footrace held in the school gym and handled himself creditably, not coming in first but ahead of two of his friends. The gym teacher kidded him and asked Rob if he had eaten frogs' legs for breakfast.

"I could go on forever discussing Rob's improvements and successes, both big and small. I must also add that when he is off his medication on weekends, his old problems and difficulties return in full force. By

Sunday evening his coordination and disorganization are very bad: He falls against the furniture and bumps into walls. In fact, one Saturday night Rob got out of bed and fell against the bedpost and broke his nose. Whenever the medication is changed or accidentally forgotten, I receive a call from the teacher along the lines of 'Rob had a bad day; it was difficult to get him to settle down and do his work. He was disorganized' or 'He kept bumping into the other children.'

"At the end of the first semester, our son's report card reflected improved grades in all subjects. Three of his teachers wrote him letters in which they congratulated him upon his newfound success in speech, in reading, and in the classroom! In fact, Rob's remarkable progress has become the source of much discussion among parents and teachers. We've received many inquiries about Dr. Levinson and his diagnostic and treatment techniques.

"Four months after treatment had begun, we all experienced a new 'high,' especially Rob. He had just completed his first novel of 125 pages—in only two days! Rob was so excited about his accomplishment that he promised to read a book each week, circumstances permitting (no vacations or family/holiday outings). He has stuck to his word.

"Also, he no longer needs to track with a finger while he reads.

"Other positive developments we noticed were:

● Rob's penmanship has gotten better. Originally he drew his letters, but now he uses cursive script, and his lettering is both even and fluent.

● Rob is in the school band, playing sax. At one time his participation would have been unthinkable!

● His schoolwork and reports showed steady, consistent improvement. His classroom teacher said that at the beginning of the school year she was very satisfied with good effort and a few good papers a week. For Rob to complete his work at all was truly an accomplishment. However, in May, the end of the school year, Rob's teacher reported that she never received less than A- or B-quality material from him—quite astounding, not only to his teacher, but to us as well! We are so proud of him that there are no words that can possibly convey our feelings.

● Rob shows a real flair for arts and crafts, the discovery of which was an unexpected bonus. Several of his creations were chosen to go on display in the school showcase. On the strength of his contributions, he was chosen to participate in the Gifted Art Program offered by the school for the next year.

"Rob still tires easily upon occasion, but he does not get wiped out the way he did before treatment. Also, he experiences reversals, but these occur *less and less frequently*. School days that are particularly hectic with extra activities are difficult for him—the less confusion, the better. He is also able to function well in small groups. Before, he could only do so on a one-to-one basis. Family gatherings on holidays were never really enjoyable for any of us because Rob would become physically ill from the confusion, noise, and distraction. Today we all enjoy them, particularly Rob!

"Our entire family circle was dominated by the problem of having to deal with the many personnel in the educational system. We worried that Rob would be unjustly classified as retarded or pushed into delinquency by complete frustration. We all benefited from having Rob see Dr. Levinson. We were lucky that the medication brought about such good changes for our son—in the nick of time. But even more important, in understanding the root of Rob's learning disabilities, all our lives have been turned around.

"Last, but by no means least, has been the great improvement in his feelings about himself. I have tried to deal only with absolutes in listing Rob's triumphs and accomplishments. There have been many other positive, noticeable, more subtle changes that relate to Rob's attitudes, self-esteem, and sense of well-being that I have not included but are very much a part of this year's success story."

In a progress report in 1982, Mrs. Stone glowingly wrote about Rob's year in the fourth grade, a school year characterized by the same wonderful and positive results in his academic and behavior performances.

Dr. Levinson's program of treatment and follow-up, good teacher support, Rob's self-determination, and the guidance of a loving reading teacher contributed to the transformation of a floundering, unhappy young child to a much talked about, successful, happy youngster.

The early years of life are the most formative, shaping the personality, behavior, and values of young people. The influence of the school upon the child, like that of the family, is immeasurable. That influence has the potential for both good and bad, depending upon the individuals in the educational structure, their qualifications, and their predilections to be fair, open-minded, and responsive to the needs of children. Educators and counselors with whom a child is in daily contact, and the positive and negative experiences in the school and classroom, determine, in large measure, how the child views himself and how he views others—his parents, siblings, teachers, and peers. This, in turn, influences his behavior and attitudes, facilitating or hindering a successful and happy adjustment to his world scholastically, personally, and socially.

The two school systems depicted in the story of Rob Stone and his family thought they were caring and responsive. One was just beginning to deal with children who have learning disorders. However, it was antiquated and not sufficiently knowledgeable in its approach. Had the Stones followed its proposal, their son would have been placed in a school for brain-damaged children, probably resulting in emotional scarring.

Upon returning to visit friends in the community in which they had lived, the Stones learned that four families had removed their children from the same school for reasons similar to theirs. The school did not have the program or facilities to deal effectively with children who had learning disabilities. Their staff was limited in its thinking and lacked the open-mindedness and flexibility needed to explore different concepts and theories. Fortunately the Stones and the other four families recognized the deficits in the school before emotional fallout and other consequences permanently damaged their children. Unfortunately there were other families who did follow the recommendations of the school.

On the other hand, the second school system, which was similar in size and population, did have a program for learning-disabled children and had qualified personnel to execute it. However, their personnel's knowledge and diagnostic techniques were incomplete and, in some instances, biased. They were victims, in a way, of their own "dyslexia"— blind to the problems of those children who did not fit the "pattern," who did not conform to their psychoeducational theories.

Just as this chapter was being completed, in walked Dr. Larry A. Sternson, Professor of Pharmaceutical Chemistry at the University of Kansas's College of Pharmacy, with his son, Tom. They had come for a revisit. He expressed his delight with Tom's progress and discussed some of the problems he experienced with members of the educational system. With his permission I am including some of his important comments:

> Some educators are reluctant to learn, to read, and to change their opinions as to how children with dyslexia should be treated. It is easier to blame parents, environmental situations, and other factors, and to conclude with the statement that "if the little guy would just buckle down, we know that he would succeed." They seem unable to grasp that the inability to buckle down is a direct manifestation of the disorder and is not controllable. . . .

Inasmuch as some critics have attributed the favorable responses of my patients to "the placebo effect," at the end of our clinical visit I jokingly asked Professor Sternson what he thought of his son's remarkable response to the "placebo" treatment I had prescribed. He replied:

There is no way in the world a placebo effect could produce such dramatic and long-lasting effects in a child, especially a child unfamiliar with the effects of medication. No other therapy I have ever offered to Tom has had a placebo effect. He has been to optometrists, occupational therapists, and special educators, and he has never had an effect like this before. Surely his mother, he, and I all wanted the same response effect from the beginning. Moreover he responded better to certain medications than to others, and not at all to one.

And when we took him off the medication on weekends, his symptoms came back again after two days and lasted until Tuesday or Wednesday of the following week. We had to rearrange the manner in which we took him off the medication to avoid this effect.

How is my son to psychologically know when the medication effect wears off and then begins again?

It is very obviously a medication effect—a true medication effect.

Although many educators and school psychologists believe only *they* have the understanding and the knowledge of the dynamics of child development and the educational process, this is not true. More and more parents are knowledgeable, aware, and anxious to participate in this process. The children can only benefit if these two most important and powerful forces combine their strengths to achieve their common goal: helping each child fulfill his own potential to become all he has the capacity to be.

Obviously not all school systems are like the two depicted in the story of the Stone family. There are others whose professionalism, objectivity, and open-mindedness about new ideas and proven concepts are supportive to both the dyslexic child and his family. I hope this chapter serves to enlighten further and to enlarge the numbers of such school systems.

7
A Deaf Girl
Can Hear Clearly

ONE OF THE MOST REMARKABLE CASES I HAVE THUS FAR
treated is that of Consuelo Brody, a lovely, highly intelligent young lady
of seventeen years. What makes Consuelo's story unique is that she was
either born deaf or became deaf shortly after birth. Later, at the age of
seventeen, she had her hearing significantly restored by using the very
same medications I use with dyslexics. Today Consuelo's hearing is so
much better that she can attend a college for "normal" children instead
of a special school that compensates for the hearing-impaired.

How this truly remarkable story came about and the uniqueness of
Consuelo's case might be the subject of a program such as *That's Incredible*. It illustrates the unexpected relationship between deafness and dyslexia, and highlights the important ramifications of this correlation.

It was Consuelo's deafness that motivated her mother to delve into the
study of hearing loss. She was determined to do all she could to help her
daughter overcome this handicap. Accordingly, Mrs. Brody became a
speech and hearing specialist.

Consuelo's deafness was not typical. Her mother noticed two episodes
in which her daughter appeared to hear despite having been diagnosed
as severely hearing-impaired.

The first incident occurred at the time Consuelo was two years old.
Mrs. Brody related the following:

I put the new baby's bottle to my mouth and said "Bottle, bottle." Consuelo looked at me and put her finger into her ear, pulled it out, and said "Bott." She repeated it. I couldn't believe it! Consuelo had never repeated a word in her life up to that point.

A couple of years later the second incident occurred. Consuelo was in the bathtub. Outside the bathroom her sister, Denise, was playing the harmonica. Suddenly, Consuelo put her finger in her ear, smiled, and uttered the sound "Ahh!" She had obviously heard the sound and she was not wearing her hearing aid. I asked Denise to continue to play so that I could observe Consuelo's reactions. Every time Denise began to play, Consuelo would put her finger into her ear and smile. She had heard! I was so excited!

Consuelo knew about twenty-five words. I covered my mouth and repeated these words. She then repeated them, getting every word right! I was stunned! An hour later I said the words once again in a similar manner, but this time Consuelo did not hear anything. I could not understand how this occurred. I had to find out what was wrong!

Mrs. Brody read through book after book in order to understand how her deaf child could episodically hear. She stumbled upon a disorder called Ménière's disease, one that causes an adult to lose his hearing acuity and impairs his balance and coordination system, i.e., his inner-ear system.

Mrs. Brody wondered: "Could my daughter have had Ménière's disease since birth? Could that explain why her hearing appeared to deteriorate with age, and account for the episodes in which her hearing came and went?"

While taking speech and hearing classes, Mrs. Brody consulted many teachers. Some were sympathetic, but they all said the same thing: "How could a child have Ménière's disease?"

Two additional unexplained but related episodes helped convince Mrs. Brody that her daughter indeed had Ménière's disease. One morning, when Consuelo was six years old, she was standing perfectly still and suddenly fell forward. Consuelo had apparently momentarily lost all balance control.

When seven and a half years of age, Consuelo was seated in the living room and suddenly, very calmly, drew a circular motion with her hand and repeatedly said "Round." Following this motion, she stood up and appeared to stagger across the room, unable to climb the stairs. A few minutes after this episode, she was back to normal.

These two episodes of imbalance and dizziness convinced Mrs. Brody that her intuition and theory regarding her daughter were accurate. She consulted a famous ear, nose, and throat specialist. The following are excerpts from his consultation report, supporting Mrs. Brody's conclusion.

There are a number of factors that make it a most unusual case. . . . I do not believe that Connie's hearing loss is of a congenital nature but due to some abnormality in the inner ear. This may explain the occasional return of good hearing, the tinnitus and recurrent vertigo and imbalance.

This is a most unusual situation and I feel that every effort should be made to improve her hearing on a conservative basis.

She also consulted a neurologist. However, this specialist was skeptical of Mrs. Brody's observations, due to the fact that she was both a mother and a specialist in hearing and speech. Thus, he states, "This has raised a suspicion of overenthusiasm concerning the reported signs and symptoms. . . . If, indeed, Consuelo has had dizzy episodes and remarkable spontaneous episodes of improved hearing, then an end-organ (ear) disease causing profound deafness should be seriously suspected. However, one must be very cautious. . . ."

It is interesting and sad how bias can sidestep crucial observations because they were made by a mother who also happened to be a specialist in the very area she was observing. Again, bias confused fact for fantasy, and the burden of what to do was dumped back on the parent.

Fortunately, Mrs. Brody made the correct decision. She took her daughter to see a famous neuro-otologist—a surgeon specializing in correcting deficits within the ear and the inner-ear system. He confirmed Mrs. Brody's suspicions and operated on Consuelo.

This surgery appeared successful in arresting further hearing deterioration. "But," wondered Mrs. Brody, "what would have happened if I had taken Connie to this doctor when she was an infant? Had he operated on her at that time, could this surgery have kept her hearing from getting so much worse?"

Following Mrs. Brody's visit to the specialist and prior to Connie's surgery, a trial of an antihistamine was advised. Mrs. Brody noted an improvement in her daughter's hearing discrimination. However, upon retesting her audiologically, the doctor did not find any change.

Only in retrospect did Mrs. Brody stumble upon the reason for the discrepancy in her observation and the doctor's testing. In reality, both pieces of paradoxical observations were correct.

The doctor had tested Connie with individual "beep" tones, a test to evaluate auditory acuity. Mrs. Brody on the other hand, observed an improvement in Connie's ability to discriminate spoken sounds. Her testing revealed an improvement in her auditory discrimination.

Indeed, Connie's hearing acuity had not improved on the antihistamine. Thus, her scores when tested with "beeps" did not change while using the medication. However, Mrs. Brody's testing was also correct. Her auditory discrimination had significantly improved, and the reasons for this discrepancy will be described shortly.

Connie also exhibited another interesting and seemingly paradoxical symptom: Her ability to read lips was significantly worse when wearing her hearing aid. This observation was corroborated by all. Mrs. Brody stated, "I noticed that when her hearing aid was on, she would say 'What? What?' then, when the hearing aid was turned off, she understood me. Needless to say, this is a most unusual reaction. Generally, when one wears a hearing aid and does lip-reading, one's comprehension is much better. Lip reading and use of a hearing aid tend to complement one another. But with Consuelo the opposite was true. She became more confused."

Although Consuelo's hearing had stopped deteriorating, the picture she presented to her parents was not only confusing but bleak. While vacationing, Mrs. Brody happened to be watching *Donahue!* in 1982. She reports: "I almost fell out of my seat because Dr. Levinson began to talk about the prescription drug Meclizine and its importance in treating people with dyslexia, describing how it improved their reading and how the inner-ear system and its computer, the cerebellum, acts as a mediator between the senses and the higher centers in the brain."

Mrs. Brody ran to the library and read *A Solution to the Riddle Dyslexia* from cover to cover. She suddenly understood all the paradoxical observations of her daughter. She suddenly understood why her daughter's hearing acuity had not improved with the medication, whereas her auditory discrimination had: "Suddenly, I began to see it all very clearly. It was almost like a revelation. A revolutionary discovery had been made within the speech and audiology fields."

Connie's auditory acuity did not really improve on the medication. That's all the "beeps" tested for. However, she did improve in her ability to discriminate *sounds* and sound sequences in sentences. In other words, the medicine helped her inner-ear system better fine-tune the sound sequences coming into the brain. Accordingly she could better discriminate them, despite the fact that her hearing acuity did not change. That is to say, Connie had two problems: an auditory acuity problem that did not respond to medication, and a dyslexic disorder secondary to a dysfunction within her inner-ear system. Her total hearing was a result of two factors, hearing acuity and the ability to distinguish sound sequences. By treating the latter factor, Connie's overall ability to hear words and sentences had indeed improved.

If the auditory input is not properly fine-tuned, it is received by the thinking brain as blurry, just as visual signals are. The medication tends to fine-tune the auditory input, thus helping words become increasingly clear and comprehensible.

Mrs. Brody brought Connie to my office August 1982. After appropriate testing, I noted that Connie indeed had dyslexia. This diagnosis also cleared up the last remaining confusing observation: why Connie couldn't read lips and use a hearing aid at the same time. Dyslexics frequently have difficulty coordinating two or more functions simultaneously.

Connie was placed back on the prescription drug Meclizine as well as a series of other vitamins and medication. Today she is remarkedly improved. Her auditory discrimination has dramatically increased from about 15 percent to about 65 to 70 percent using a hearing aid. This means that she can function in a world of normal hearing.

Connie's medication has also helped solve another very difficult problem associated with Ménière's disease: recruitment. Recruitment is a phenomenon that occurs when the volume or amplitude of the hearing aid is turned up. Suddenly there is the mushrooming surge of sounds that fuzzes and confuses the incoming signals, rendering discrimination difficult, even impossible.

With the medication, however, Consuelo can now increase the amplitude of her hearing aid without the occurrence of high-frequency distortion or screeching. The medication enables her to filter out selectively or inhibit background and even mushrooming noises, thus greatly improving her ability to use a hearing aid effectively. These observations and discoveries have added a whole new dimension to the treatment of Ménière's disease and related hearing losses in which there exists a hidden disturbance within the inner-ear system.

For many years Consuelo had been having her hearing tested by audiologist Dr. Harvey J. Gardner (Director, Huntington Hearing & Speech Center and former Director of Audiology, Manhattan Eye, Ear & Throat Hospital). Her test on July 27, 1982, showed an auditory discrimination (clarity of heard words) score of 16 percent in her better ear. While she was on medication Dr. Gardner conducted a series of retests until on October 19, 1982, her score jumped to 52 percent, a fantastic improvement. Even more important, on March 14, 1983, her binaural score climbed to 60 percent, up from 12 percent in earlier testing. Now, she could integrate information heard in both ears! Mrs. Brody also took her daughter to visit the surgeon who had operated on her in 1977. His testing further substantiated that of the new doctor. A fantastic improvement was noted: Her auditory discrimination jumped from 0 to 32 percent. The second score was slightly less than the first only because the second doctor used recordings, which tend to distort the sound slightly, whereas the first doctor's testing was with the live voice. However, both groups of tests showed the same results: a 32-percent differential and improvement without the use of a hearing aid.

For the very first time a deaf patient with Ménière's disease could hear with a hearing aid as a result of a simple medical treatment.

Consuelo is now a much happier, more confident, more outgoing young lady. On the Stamford Reading Achievement Test, her scores indicated that she had jumped five years in one, a jump never seen before at her school. Consuelo's visual and auditory senses are now in harmony, complementing and catalyzing one another. Moreover, her improvement extends to other areas: math, biology—indeed, all her other subjects. She is now scoring at the top of her class in almost all subjects. She is able to understand and enjoy watching TV. For the first time in her life she will go to stores alone and shop. Consuelo's success story is remarkable, not only from the medical-scientific point of view, but also from her own inner "feeling" point of view. Entirely new vistas will now open to a previously deaf child, enabling her to explore and appreciate *all* the beauty and wonder that is a part of life for a normal, healthy youngster. Her life and feelings have been rekindled and further awakened.

For Mrs. Brody, there resulted an answer to her determination, dedication, and prayers.

Connie's life is now open-ended for the first time ever. She is no longer restricted and confined by her severe hearing and dyslexic disability. She can become anything she desires.

However, there is more to this story. As a result of Consuelo's significant improvement, her brother Fred, age sixteen, and sister Marie, age fifteen, were also brought to me for examination and treatment. Both Marie and Fred had attended the Learning Disability Unit of Adelphi University for five years, but their progress was minimal. Both had superior IQs but were having trouble in school. Both had difficulties with reading, spelling, and concentration, and both had experienced words as blurry. Consuelo, on the other hand, had experienced sounds as blurry. Inasmuch as Marie's blurred vision bothered her significantly, she was examined by an optometrist, who found her eyes to be in normal condition. Unfortunately, glasses did not help.

Of the two children, Fred seemed to have the more severe problem. Although he had a high IQ and an inquisitive mind, Fred was unable to sit still or concentrate on anything for more than a few moments. His grades were not good and he hardly spoke, appearing to be very much an introvert. He was neither verbally dull nor schizoid. He just found it very difficult to verbalize his thoughts, even with his family. Consequently he withdrew, finding it much easier to listen than to speak.

Both Fred and Marie were diagnosed as dyslexic, and after evaluation and treatment, both children showed marked improvement.

Despite extra help, Marie had been a C student. She now receives grades in the nineties in math, social studies, and biology. During tests, her teachers now seat her at the back of the room to be sure no one copies from her.

Fred is now getting A's in math and chemistry and B's in his other subjects. His reading, grammar, spelling, and sentence structure are so improved that his already amazed family feel even more amazed. His writing appears normal; he is more verbal and is now an active participant rather than a silent, introverted observer.

This family of dyslexic individuals highlights the already-known fact that dyslexia can be inherited. (Mr. Brody is dyslexic as well.) But although multiple family members may have the very same underlying disorder, both the intensity and combination of symptoms may vary significantly from one family member to another. Thus, family members who are normal readers but have only mild writing, spelling, mathematical, or directional disturbances most often do not realize they have dyslexia. Researchers who do not detect family members with normal reading problems often make a similar mistake. As a result, most statistics having to do with genetic dyslexia have been subject to significant degrees of errors.

8

Solving the Dyslexic Riddle—A Historical Perspective

AFTER HAVING BEEN EXPOSED TO A RATHER LARGE SAMPLE of dyslexic patients, to their symptoms, experiences, and responses to treatment, as well as to my latest concept of the dyslexic disorder, the reader may find this belated presentation of history after the fact, out of joint—indeed, reversed.

Do not be thrown by this reversal. Indeed, dyslexics frequently use their unstable directional and reversal mechanisms to significant advantage. And I have attempted to learn from them what I can. By shifting the history of my research effort from the beginning to the end of this book, I have given the reader time, experience, and perspective. I hope this dyslexialike organizational device will prove immensely helpful.

The ability to reverse flexibly, backtrack, and change directions has indeed been immeasurably helpful to me in guiding my research effort to a sound conclusion. Most often, research does not proceed along a straight line. Clues suddenly appear and disappear and even twist into elusive arcs. Researchers must be able to adapt to these rapidly shifting and directed flashes.

In many ways I felt my research techniques oscillating between the typical behavior of Oscar and Felix in TV's famed *Odd Couple*. Interestingly, both Oscar and Felix reflect the extreme variations characterizing the dyslexic disorder. For example, Oscar's disorganization highlights the underlying dyscoordination, whereas Felix represents its overcompensatory extreme, reflecting a rigid need to control one's underlying chaos by developing rigid personality controls. Although the discipline symbolized by Felix is crucial to any research endeavor, this discipline must be viewed as an aid rather than the burden of compulsive rigidity hampering Felix. Therefore, I have attempted to escape the restrictions imposed by a Felix-like mental and scientific rigor mortis by choosing a flexible, "dyslexialike" (as opposed to "normal") sequential writing style.

Having completed this introductory apology, I will now relate to you the path leading me to resolve the riddle characterizing dyslexia and my dyslexic research.

My "dyslexic" career began entirely by chance some twenty years ago. I had just completed my psychiatric residency and sought an interesting position that might help support me economically while I began a private practice in psychiatry. A new position suddenly appeared at the Bureau of Child Guidance (BCG, New York City Board of Education). Psychiatrists were needed to treat the many children experiencing learning, emotional, and behavioral difficulties within the New York City educational system.

By chance I was assigned to a tiny bureau within this giant educational complex, the Bureau of Special Reading Services (SRS). Children within this special reading tutorial service were accepted only if: (1) they were two or more years behind their peers in reading, (2) they had a normal or above normal IQ, (3) they were not disruptive or behavior problems, and (4) they had no evidence of brain damage or any type of sensory defect. Only later did I realize that the acceptance criteria of the SRS were identical to the criteria utilized by most experts to define dyslexics.

In any event the prevailing opinion within this clinically oriented tutorial service was that reading disabilities were caused by psychological factors. Accordingly the clinical team examining children consisted of a specially trained reading teacher, a social worker, a psychologist, and a psychiatrist.

Every child within the SRS received two hours of tutoring a week in very small groups. And each child received a complete social work and psychological workup. Only those children failing to benefit significantly from the tutoring were seen and treated psychiatrically.

Having been trained psychiatrically, and having had little experience with the reading-disabled, I had no question or quarrel with the psychological point of view of the SRS. Indeed, I read through all the available psychiatric and psychoanalytical theories linking reading disorders with such emotional causes as sibling rivalry, competitive difficulties, fear of success, child-rearing difficulties (abuses and/or pampering and overpampering), sexual and/or aggressive fantasies having to do with looking or the eye, Oedipal conflicts, classroom abuse, etc.

Thus, over a period of many years, I came to examine psychiatrically and later neurologically over a thousand reading-disabled children coming from all socioeconomic and cultural areas of New York City. Diligently, I attempted to apply all existing psychological and analytical theories and principles when analyzing and treating the reading-disabled children psychotherapeutically. After a number of years of painstaking effort, I reluctantly concluded that a vast majority of psychological theories attempting to explain the causes and symptoms of reading disabilities had little to do with the cases I saw. The many symptoms characterizing the reading-disabled and the psychological theories attempting to explain them just did not correlate despite all my determined attempts to link them together. Reluctantly, I was eventually forced to wonder:

• Was I personally inadequate in applying psychological theories espoused by respected analysts to the reading disorders I examined, or
• Was it possible that my respected teachers and researchers were inadequately espousing theories that had little or nothing to do with clinical reality?

Although personally I felt inclined to blame myself, and repeatedly did so, I eventually came to recognize that the vast majority of reading-disabled children and their families just did not fit into the psychologically accepted molds. Existing psychological theories could neither explain the cause of reading disorders for the vast majority of children I examined nor explain the typical reading and related symptoms characterizing the learning-disabled.

It is easy to understand how researchers originally formed the conviction that the reading and academic disturbances in dyslexia were of a primary psychological origin. Do not dyslexics and the learning-disabled feel dumb, ugly, and hopeless? Are these not psychological symptoms? Are not dyslexic individuals prone to emotional and behavioral disorders, as well as a series of phobias, obsessions and compulsions, mood disturbances, and even psychosomatic symptoms such as bed-wetting, muscle tics, headaches, dizziness, nausea, vomiting, and abdominal pain? Are not these symptoms typically those that fall within the psychiatric and psychological realms and spheres of influence?

However, if the theory does not clinically and statistically fit the facts, the theory must be in error. It sounds simple to say this now but it was not easy to detach myself from theories and convictions I'd lived with for years. Old established scientific theories seldom fade away. They are clung to like religious symbols, even when defying all new scientific realities.

Scientific frustration and clinical despair can be handled in two ways. You can either start over or sidestep the whole conflict by initially denying the existence of fallacious theories based on created or fantasized data.

Starting over appears easy and exciting only in hindsight. In the beginning it is a lonely, time-consuming, frustrating experience. And only those with an intense curiosity and/or a low frustration tolerance are appropriately motivated to leap into new and unsanctioned scientific spheres.

Patients and teachers needed help. And I needed a scientific theory and concept I could live with and hang my hat on. I needed a way of helping my patients and their families, a way to justify my many years of training.

I began to search out other theories in my attempt to explain the causes and symptoms of learning disabilities and dyslexia. Because of my medical background, it seemed only reasonable for me to assume that dyslexia had to be of a neurological origin if it were not psychologically based.

The prevailing neurological theory at the time was that dyslexia and its related symptoms were due to a disturbance within the thinking, speaking, IQ brain—the cerebral cortex. Ever since Kerr and Morgan* first recognized and described "word blindness" in 1896, it was assumed and believed that this disorder was due to a structural defect within the dominant half of the thinking brain—the side of the brain responsible for recognizing written symbols and seen objects, the side of the brain responsible for and determining meaningful speech functioning and handedness.

In the vast majority of right-handed individuals, the left side of the thinking brain is crucial or dominant in determining perceptual and speech functioning. Thus, the conviction developed that an impairment of the left side of the thinking brain was responsible for dyslexia. This conviction was based upon the following assumption: *If, indeed, damage to the dominant half of the thinking brain is proven responsible for the loss of reading and speech ability in previously normal adults via autopsy stud-*

*See p. 1.

ies, then children suffering from reading and/or speech disorders must have an impairment in this very same area of the brain.

The basis of this scientifically irresistible neurological theory is still held in wide esteem, albeit in slightly modified forms. However, there was an obvious flaw in this theory. Inasmuch as there currently exists no clinical evidence of cerebral damage in dyslexia, and in view of the fact that many *bright,* even gifted, children and adults had and have dyslexia, it seemed reasonable to assume that there was really nothing structurally wrong with the thinking brain. As a result, many neurologists assumed that the dominant brain was intact, but that its development was *delayed.*

This watered-down version of cerebral damage and dysfunction was more in harmony with the facts although it still did not explain *all* or even a fragment of the data. And most unfortunately it could not be proven. This theory *had* to be accepted as is, without validation. Clinicians were taught and expected to dance to the traditional scientific tune. And resistance to any challenge and change was—and still is—intense.

Interestingly, an alternative hypothesis was denied: If, indeed, a cerebral developmental lag or delay was present, and if, in addition, there was no clear-cut clinical evidence of any cerebral dysfunction, might not the searched-for disturbance be caused by a dysfunction in a noncortical area of the brain—a dysfunction secondarily causing this cerebral lag or delay? No cortically based investigator attempted to search for the root of dyslexia in noncerebral cortical areas of the brain.

Some neurologists believe that dyslexia is due to a *lack* of dominance of one half of the thinking brain versus its other mirrored half. This theory is based on the reasoning and findings of a gifted psychiatrist-neurologist, Samuel Orton. Orton correlated dyslexia with speech disorders and a high incidence of left-handedness, and renamed the disorder *strephosymbolia,* meaning twisted symbols. He based his cerebral dominance theory and conviction on the following reasoning:

- If, indeed, the dominant half of the cerebral cortex, or the thinking brain, controls reading and speech functions as well as right-handedness, and
- If cases with reading disorders have a higher incidence of speech disorders and left-handedness than they should have when compared with normal individuals,
- Then there must be a *lack* of dominance or control of the left-thinking brain.
- Moreover, this lack of left-sided dominance results in a *dominance conflict,* or dyscoordination, between the two halves of the cerebral cortex, resulting in reversals.

Although this dominance theory was interesting, it had many drawbacks. The most crucial drawback was one that Orton himself later recognized—that one of his basic assumptions was wrong: Dyslexia does *not* occur more often in left-handed individuals.

In addition the speech disturbances noted in dyslexia are of a type found only in disorders of balance and coordination, i.e., inner-ear–related disorders. They are not of cerebral origin (the aphasic type)—speech disturbances in which individuals have difficulty understanding the meaning of what is said and/or difficulty in formulating the meaning of what they wish to say. Thus, I concluded, Orton's second assumption was also wrong. The speech disorders in dyslexia are not of a type due to a dysfunction within the thinking brain.

In addition, the cerebral dominance theory of dyslexia suffers from the same drawbacks that negate the cerebral-lag theory of dyslexia:

- There is no way to prove or disprove the dominance theory of dyslexia.
- Its basic assumptions were found to be in error.
- It cannot explain the vast majority of symptoms in dyslexia.
- It has led nowhere diagnostically or therapeutically—medically.
- An alternative explanation was never considered: that if indeed there were dyscoordinated and conflicting dominance of the two hemispheres, this difficulty might be caused by a disturbance elsewhere, namely the inner-ear system.

Despite all the above drawbacks, the dominance theory of dyslexia still has its believers and followers.

To date, the cortical theorists of dyslexia view the findings and results of optometrists, occupational therapists, etc., with suspicion. They reason as follows: If indeed dyslexia is a disturbance of the thinking, speaking, IQ part of the brain, how in the world can eye exercises, physical exercises, vitamins, diet, and medication improve the functioning of the thinking brain?

Once again, these cortical theorists have failed to view an alternative viewpoint: If eye therapy, occupational therapy, vitamins, diet and medication improve the functioning of dyslexics, and if these therapies do not primarily improve the functioning of the thinking brain, then might not dyslexia be caused by a disturbance in a noncortical area of the brain? A recent finding has created ecstasy among "cerebral cortical" followers. Autopsy studies on one assumed "dyslexic" brain revealed the presence of abnormal cells in the dominant thinking brain. Unfortunately, similar

studies were not done on the noncerebral parts of the brain—certainly
not the inner-ear system and the cerebellum. Why not? Might not a
primary disturbance within the inner-ear system and cerebellum result in
secondary disturbances within the cerebral cortex, or thinking brain?
Might not this disturbance result in impaired cellular function and an
ensuing cerebral lag?

Perhaps another example would help the reader more fully understand
the difference between a primary site of dysfunction and a secondary
reaction to it. Consider a plant and a primary disturbance within its root
system. Would not this root disturbance affect the coloring and the microscopic picture of the leaves? Most certainly! After carefully examining
the leaves, should we conclude that the disturbance in the leaf is responsible for the disturbance of the plant, especially if its roots are never
looked at?

Should we not weigh the available data appropriately? If, indeed, I
found well over 96 percent of my more than 10,000 dyslexic cases to
have evidence of an inner-ear dysfunction—and if this theory led me to
new methods of diagnosis, treatment, and a comprehensive explanation
of all the symptoms characterizing this disorder—why should one case
in which there exists cellular abnormalities within the cerebral cortex
result in overenthusiasm, especially if the cortical theories led nowhere
scientifically for the past eighty-five years?

In an attempt to harmonize this apparent "cortical" exception with my
inner-ear dyslexic rule, I wondered if the reported dyslexic patient whose
brain was studied was not a *mixed dyslexic*—a dyslexic having inner-ear
dysfunction mixed in with other evidence of brain dysfunction. If my
assumption was correct, it would explain both the exception and the rule.

I then reviewed the findings of Drs. Albert Galaburda and Thomas
Kemper reported in *Annals of Neurology* 6:94–100 (1979), entitled "Cytoarchitectonic Abnormalities in Developmental Dyslexia: A Case Study."
Interestingly this patient was reported to have developed "nocturnal sei-
zures at 16 years," a symptom unrelated to dyslexia and frequently highlighting an underlying *cerebral* dysfunction. As the authors state in this
article: "It is not possible to tell from a single case whether or not the
anatomical findings have any causative relationship to the clinical findings, much less whether the malformation is responsible for the seizure
disorder, the learning disability, both, or neither." Interestingly, cortical
theorists continue to use this single case study to "prove" their unprovable
theories, in spite of the overwhelming evidence I have amassed. Moreover, this *single* case of unproven dyslexia has been reported in the media

by cortical theorists *as if the cause and site of dyslexia may have been found.**

Instead of attempting to understand and explain this *single* case study in its proper scientific perspective, an unwarranted and overenthusiastic response is both promoted and publicized.

I always find psychological overreactions suspicious.

Over a period of many years I became as disillusioned with the prevailing neurological theories of dyslexia as I had with the psychiatric ones. Upon analysis, I concluded that both psychiatric and neurological theories, and the alleged "evidence" used to suport them, were a mixture of fact, fantasy, and fiction, with less fact than fiction. I came to view the dyslexic disorder and its research as a riddle defying all attempts at meaningful understanding, explanation, diagnosis, treatment, and prevention. This riddle, however, was scientifically solved and its existence explained in *A Solution to the Riddle Dyslexia*. For ease of presentation I will quickly summarize the steps leading to this solution.

Having been reluctantly forced to abandon the prevailing psychiatric and neurological theories, and finding all other co-existing theories limited in their explanatory scope and diagnostic-therapeutic efficacy, I sought to find the elusive cause of dyslexia and its symptomatic array.

I carefully reevaluated and analyzed all the available data, objectively searching for the hidden clues. I reviewed my own data very carefully and, to my dismay, I realized that 750 out of 1,000 consecutively examined dyslexic cases showed distinct evidence of some difficulty with balance and coordination. Only 1 percent of the cases exhibited evidence suggesting a possible cortical dysfunction.

---

*The following is an excerpt from an article entitled "Wen Smart Kids Cant Lern" by Nancy Rubin and appeared in the February 1984 issue of *Ladies' Home Journal:*

Other scientists are looking for answers in the cellular structure of the brain. Recently, neurology professor Albert Galaburda of Harvard Medical School and Dr. Thomas Kemper of Boston City Hospital conducted landmark research on the brain of a dyslexic man who died in an accident. While the brain appeared perfectly normal to the naked eye, microscopic examination of thin slices of the brain revealed a general immaturity in the structure of the left side of the brain as well as in the cells of its language centers. The doctors found gray-matter cells in parts of the brain usually containing white matter, as well as a disordered arrangement of nerve cells in the cortex, or brain covering.

As a result of such findings, Drs. Galaburda and Kemper have concluded that profound differences may exist in the brains of dyslexics, which may be the result of some chemical abnormality during an early stage of fetal development. Such chemical aberrations, says Dr. Galaburda, may have a genetic component, which would explain why dyslexia tends to run in families.

In other words my case histories indicated that the vast majority of dyslexic children demonstrated one or more of the following:

• Delayed ability to sit, crawl, walk, and/or talk
• Difficulty skipping, hopping, running, and/or participating in sports
• Fine motor coordination disturbances, such as difficulty tying shoelaces, buttoning buttons, zippering, holding a pencil, using crayons, coloring within guidelines, and/or awkward use of a knife and fork
• Dyscoordinated speech functioning, i.e., slurring, articulation impairments, stuttering, and/or stammering
• Difficulty with balance and coordination, evidenced in delays in learning to ride a bike or walk a balance beam.

Moreover, neurological examination revealed a series of clear-cut balance, coordination, and rhythmic signs consistent with the above difficulties and diagnostic of an inner-ear–system dysfunction.

As stated earlier, only 1 percent of cases showed evidence of a dysfunction within the thinking brain, i.e., low IQ, difficulty with comprehending and formulating meaningful speech, left- or right-sided weakness indicative of an earlier paralysis, epilepsy, etc.

Inasmuch as the vast majority of dyslexics revealed hard and fast evidence of dysfunctions within their inner-ear systems, despite my primary search for signs of dysfunction of the thinking brain, I was logically forced to conclude that dyslexia correlated only with inner-ear signs and not with any cortical signs.

Even researchers and clinicians believing that dyslexia was of a cerebral cortical origin found only balance and coordination (inner-ear) signs in the cases they examined. They concluded, however, that the presence of noncortical balance and coordination signs indicated that there must be something wrong with the brain. And since there were reading difficulties present, then there *had to be* a disturbance within the thinking brain, despite the complete statistical absence of cortical signs.

In other words, I believe the cortical theorists, in order to prove their theory, reasoned in circles. Their circular reasoning may be summarized as follows:

• They naturally assumed that dyslexia was of cerebral cortical origin.
• Since only inner-ear signs could be found, they termed these signs "soft" in an unconscious effort to minimize their significance.
• They further assumed that there must exist "hard" signs of cerebral dysfunction in view of the fact that "soft" signs were found, the latter (so they said) clearly suggesting the presence of a disturbance within the central nervous system.

● They concluded that dyslexia was of cerebral cortical origin and were completely satisfied that they had proved their assumption.

These cortical theorists began with an assumption that the reading disturbance in dyslexia was of cerebral cortical origin, and utilized the presence of inner-ear signs to justify the conclusion that there was a cortical dysfunction despite the fact that there were no cortical signs to be found. They then utilized the *assumption* that the reading disorder in dyslexia was of cerebral origin to conclude or prove their assumption correct.

I, too, had initially assumed that dyslexia was of cerebral cortical origin and sought to find corroborating evidence of a cerebral dysfunction. But as I found only balance and coordination difficulties—difficulties that pointed to an inner-ear dysfunction—I was forced to conclude that dyslexia is obviously not of a cerebral cortical origin and that this disorder may well be due to a dysfunction within the inner-ear system. I then conducted further clinical studies of dyslexic cases, attempting to better clarify the signs and symptoms present. These studies clearly revealed the presence of inner-ear–related disturbances 96 percent of the time. However, in these studies I was specifically looking for signs characterizing an inner-ear dysfunction. In the previous study I had been searching mainly for cortical signs, so I had found only 75 percent of the cases had evidence of an inner-ear dysfunction.

To corroborate independently my clinical findings, I sent significant samples of dyslexic cases to be examined neurologically at a major metropolitan hospital. These neurological studies also revealed that 96 percent of the cases showed signs of inner-ear dysfunction. Despite the presence of only inner-ear or cerebellar signs, these cases were frequently labeled as having minimal cerebral dysfunction or cerebral damage. Interestingly, the same hospital's neurologists invariably would label almost identical cases as having inner-ear dysfunction if the parents or children presented them with complaints of dizziness or vertigo. In other words *the neurologists frequently diagnosed their cases independently of their own clinical findings*. Restated:

● If a child complained of learning difficulties, the case was diagnosed as having "minimal cerebral dysfunction."
● If a very similar child with identical clinical findings complained of dizziness, he or she would be diagnosed as having an "inner-ear dysfunction."

These studies clearly revealed the correlation between dyslexia and inner-ear dysfunction. And in doing so they exposed the bias characterizing the interpretation of neurological data.

In addition, a rather large group of dyslexics was sent to a series of hospitals for special physiological inner-ear testing called electronystagmography (ENG). According to testing performed at New York University Medical Center, Lenox Hill Hospital, Manhattan Eye, Ear, & Throat Hospital, and Mount Sinai Hospital, 90 percent of the cases were found to show definite evidence of an inner-ear dysfunction, further confirming my own findings and even those of the first group of neurologists.

Having thus proved neurologically and physiologically that dyslexia definitely correlated with an inner-ear dysfunction, I attempted to explain how this dyslexic disorder—this sensory-input disturbance with resultant academic and intellectual dysfunctioning—can be explained on the basis of an inner-ear-related balance and coordination disturbance. Initially I reasoned as follows:

- Most dyslexics examined display eye-tracking difficulties when reading. Thus, for example, almost all dyslexic children lose their places when reading. Their eyes seem to jump wildly from letter to letter, word to word, and line to line, resulting in letter, word, and line scrambling as well as a compensatory need to guide one's eyes with a finger or card.
- The inner-ear system has been proven to direct and guide our eyes and tracking responses automatically during the reading process.
- Thus, a dysfunction of the inner ear could explain the tracking difficulties in dyslexia, and the resulting visual scrambling could explain the secondary memory, comprehension, and concentration difficulties resulting when the thinking brain receives messages that are out of sequence and/or blurry.

To prove that there truly existed tracking difficulties in dyslexics, I devised an instrument called a 3-D Optical Scanner. This instrument is capable of accurately and rapidly measuring the fixation and tracking capacity of the eye during a readinglike process.

The 3-D Optical Scanner projects a moving series of elephants (or any target), which the eyes of the tested individual are reflexively forced to follow. As the speed of the moving elephants is increased, the speed at which the eye is forced to track these accelerated elephants must correspondingly increase. Ultimately the speed of the moving elephants exceeds the ability of the eye to follow them. Blurring is then experienced; the point at which this happens is called the blurring speed.

Further testing revealed that the averge dyslexic had one-half the blurring speed or tracking capacity of nondyslexic individuals, proving that there existed an eye-tracking defect in dyslexics.

Individuals were also asked to look at a stationary sequence of elephants while a series of moving lines resembling a picket fence moved across them. Only dyslexics experienced the elephants as blurred or in movement. Nondyslexic individuals were able to fixate clearly on the stationary elephants despite the moving, overlapping background. Dyslexics' eyes would repeatedly wander off target, from foreground to background, without stability or constancy, and foreground and background were mixed and scrambled or reversed with one another.

Inasmuch as the 3-D Optical Scanner was capable of rapidly and accurately measuring eye-tracking defects, I realized it could be used as a very useful diagnostic screening instrument to detect dyslexics. Refinements in the procedure now render it more than 95 percent accurate in predicting dyslexia, and thus the presence of an underlying inner-ear dysfunction. For the very first time a medical means of detecting dyslexia had been found—an instrument independent of IQ, prior learning experiences, socio-economic factors, language barriers, and pencil-and-paper reading-and-writing tests.

Because this test was medically based and independent of reading scores, it proved highly useful in screening kindergarten children with dyslexia. Utilizing the 3-D Optical Scanner, I screened an entire kindergarten population in District 26, Queens, New York City—1,500 children. My findings revealed that approximately 20 percent of this middle-class population had dyslexia or a related underlying inner-ear dysfunction. I also demonstrated that the blurring speeds of males versus females and left-handed versus right-handed individuals were identical.

In proving that dyslexia is due to an inner-ear dysfunction, I searched for a medical means to treat this disorder. By viewing the dyslexic tracking impairment as similar to that experienced by normal individuals when reading in a car moving along a bumpy road, or while in a boat tossed by waves, or after spinning, I realized that dyslexia may also be viewed as similar to a form of motion sickness, although it is not necessarily accompanied by the nausea and vomiting that characterizes motion sickness. I therefore attempted to treat dyslexics with anti–motion-sickness medications and related pharmaceutical agents.* I reasoned that if such medications helped the inner ear handle the motion input in motion sickness, thus alleviating the motion-sickness symptoms, then these very same medications might similarly help the dyslexic reading process resulting from a dysfunctioning inner-ear system.

Fortunately testing proved the above assumptions to be correct in most

---

*Reminder: Because of possible side effects, no one should attempt to treat himself without a doctor's supervision.

cases, as the reader has already noted in Chapter IV. Initially, I expected only the reading symptoms in dyslexia to improve with medication. To my delight and surprise a whole series of sensorimotor symptoms improved, including hearing (auditory) and touch (tactile) sequencing functions.* Accordingly, I designed two new additional instruments capable of measuring auditory blurring and tactile blurring in a manner similar to the way my 3-D Optical Scanner measured visual blurring.

To measure auditory blurring, I devised an instrument capable of speeding up a series of clear sounds until they could no longer be distinguished, thus establishing the auditory blurring speed. In a similar fashion I designed another instrument capable of tapping out touch (tactile) patterns on one's arm or hand. As the pattern speed intensified, one could no longer distinguish or feel the pattern, at which time tactile blurring would result. Further experiments clearly highlighted the fact that auditory blurring and tactile blurring speeds are lower for dyslexics than they are for unimpaired individuals, just as the visual blurring speeds are lower for the former than the latter. By obtaining visual, auditory, and tactile blurring speeds, dyslexia can be better diagnosed and the corresponding sensory-processing defects better delineated.

The collection and analysis of the dyslexic treatment responses to the anti–motion-sickness medications led me to an entirely new concept of dyslexia, a concept far wider in scope and depth than my original, rather simplistic tracking hypothesis.

I realized that the dyslexic disorder reached into and affected most areas of one's waking and sleeping lives. Hence, I came to view the inner-ear system as a fine-tuner for the entire sensory-input and motor-output system. (Interestingly, I later found the above observations to be in perfect harmony with a series of animal experiments conducted by an outstanding group of neurophysiologists—R. S. Snider, A. Stowell, R. S. Dow, R. Anderson, and E. D. Adrian—one of them, Adrian, a Nobel prizewinner.)

Perhaps a quote from Ray Snider's magnificent *Scientific American* article "The Cerebellum" will highlight this "fine-tuner" theory:

> In the back of our skulls, perched upon the brain stem under the overarching mantle of the great hemispheres of the cerebrum, is a baseball-sized, bean-

---

*Many a dyslexic would hear a tune or sound sequence as blurry or partially blurry, mirroring the way in which they experienced letters and words as visibly blurred, scrambled, reversed, or moving. The same was found true for the perception of accelerated sequences of touch sensations.

shaped lump of gray and white brain tissue. This is the cerebellum, the "lesser brain". In contrast to the cerebrum, where men have sought and found the centers of so many vital mental activities, the cerebellum remains a region of subtle and tantalizing mystery, its function hidden from investigators. . . . Its elusive signals have begun to tell us that, while the cerebellum itself directs no body functions, it operates as monitor and coordinator of the brain's other centers and as mediator between them and the body. . . . As in the cerebrum, the various functions of the cerebellum are localized in distinctly defined areas of its cortex. Detection and plotting of the electrical activity of the cortex has made it possible to map these areas. The control of the body's equilibrium, for example, is localized in the extreme front and rear surfaces of the cerebellum. . . .

For a long time it was thought that . . . the cerebellum was restricted to the management of the body's equilibrium and muscular activity. However, at the Johns Hopkins University in 1942 Averill Stowell and I undertook an investigation which has established that the cerebellum is equally involved in the coordination of the sensations of touch, hearing and sight. . . .

Our investigation showed also that the tactile, visual and auditory centers of the cerebellum are linked to the corresponding centers in the cerebral cortex. . . .

. . . In sum, the cerebellar circuitry is an accessory control system imposed upon the basic ascending (sensory) and descending (motor) circuits of the nervous system. . . . One is tempted to see the cerebellum as the great "modulator" of nervous function. . . . In the meantime we may have to contend with the possibility that the cerebellum is involved in still more diverse aspects of the nervous system. It becomes increasingly evident that if "integration" is a major function of this organ, trips into the realm of mental disease may cross its boundaries more frequently than the guards in sanitariums suspect.*

Analysis of the symptoms of thousands of dyslexics, and the study of their treatment responses to medications, eventually led me to the insight that a vast number of phobias, mood and behavior disorders, "psychosomatic" symptoms, etc., are part and parcel of the dyslexic disorder. While still in psychiatric practice, I examined all my psychiatric patients for dyslexia, utilizing my 3-D Optical Scanner. Surprisingly, *all* my phobic patients were found to be dyslexic. Thus, I was forced to revamp completely the psychiatric theory of phobias and related disorders, just as I had been forced to revamp the psychiatric and neurological theories of dyslexia. Many theories, which perpetuated myths about dyslexia, corresponded to what the renowned philosopher and writer Arthur Koest-

*R. Snider, "The Cerebellum," *Scientific American*, Vol. 174 (1958), pp 84–90.

ler refers to as a "closed system" of scientific thought.* Inasmuch as a significant number of traditionally accepted neurological and psychiatric assumptions were found to be either incorrect or inadequate, and in view of the fact that these previously unquestioned and unchallenged assumptions originally guided my research's directions, it is no wonder that my efforts frequently went astray. Backtracking and beginning anew became commonplace techniques for me. However, with determination and twenty years of effort, each and every apparent dead end and paradox has been resolved. And following each resolution, I stumbled upon unexpected and undreamed-of insights—and the opening up of entirely new research vistas.

As stated in Chapter I, dyslexia was traditionally viewed as merely a severe reading disorder. In fact, many experts even demanded that dyslexics must be two or more years behind their peers in order to qualify for this diagnosis. In attempting to perfect my 3-D Optical Scanner, I tested dyslexics with severe reading disorders as well as normal individuals. These studies clearly revealed that the blurring speeds of dyslexics were half that of nondyslexics.

So far, so good.

But when a research team attempted to duplicate and extend my studies, they ran into a number of serious problems that could not be explained until several years later. This team could not clearly distinguish a foolproof correlation between severe reading disorders and low blurring speeds. In other words they found significant numbers of children with mild and even normal reading scores to have low blurring speeds. And the reverse was true as well. Not all children with low blurring speeds had severe reading disorders. In fact, some were good readers. These findings seemed impossible to me, and I was emotionally devastated and bewildered. These findings were far from predictable.

Only after several additional years of frustrating research did a simple answer materialize. *My instrument was right. The existing concept of dyslexia was wrong.*

Eventually, I found dyslexia to be significantly independent of reading

*A closed system is a cognitive structure . . . where parallels intersect and straight lines form loops. Its canon is based on a central axiom, postulate or dogma, to which the subject is emotionally committed, and from which the rules of processing reality are derived. The amount of distortion involved in the processing is a matter of degrees, and an important criterion of the value of the system. It ranges from the scientist's involuntary inclination to juggle with data as a mild form of self-deception, motivated by his commitment to a theory, to the delusional belief-systems of clinical paranoia. [Arthur Koestler, *The Ghost in the Machine* (New York: Macmillan, 1968), p. 264.]

scores—a far cry from the definition according to which dyslexics had to be two or more years behind their peers in reading tests. Several reasons were found to explain the traditional correlation between dyslexia and severe reading impairment. "Experts" saw only the severely disturbed readers, for only the most impaired were referred for expert examination. Consequently it was assumed that dyslexia occurred only in the form of a severe reading impairment.

There was another good reason for confusing and even equating dyslexics with severely impaired readers. In 1896, when dyslexia was first recognized, clinicians assumed that this disorder was similar to alexia, a total inability of previously normal adults to recognize the meaning of written symbols. Alexia occurred in normal reading adults only following a stroke or lesion of one specific area of the dominant half of the thinking brain. The clinicians therefore mistakenly assumed that the failure of dyslexic children to acquire normal reading ability resulted from a disturbance within the cerebral cortex, identical to that causing normal reading adults to lose completely their recognition of written symbols.

As natural as this assumption was, it turned out to be completely wrong. No one had properly analyzed the *quality* of the reading disturbances in alexic adults and compared it with the quality of the reading disturbances in dyslexic children. Although alexic and dyslexic individuals both have reading difficulties, the quality of the reading disturbances in the two disorders is as different as night and day.*

All dyslexics know the meanings of written symbols; it is just that they have difficulty remembering them. For example, all dyslexics know that the letter *b* is a letter, but sometimes they confuse its directional orientation. Hence, they may guess and call a *b* a *d*, or *p* a *q*. They know the word *was* is either *was* or *saw,* again highlighting a directional uncertainty, not a conceptual or symbolic disturbance.

Alexic adults look at the letter *b* and the word *saw* and haven't the foggiest idea of their respective meanings. If they guess, a *b* may be called *3,* and *was* may be called *elephant.* Inasmuch as alexic adults have difficulty recognizing the meaning of the written symbols they see, their reading disorders are invariably severe.

Dyslexics, on the other hand, can and do learn to read. They merely have difficulty doing so. Their reading difficulties are characterized by

---

*Some alexic individuals appear to display a secondary release and destabilization of interconnecting inner ear (cerebellar) circuits which result in a combined cortical–inner ear symptomatic mix. Accordingly, these cases are now under investigation.

memory and directional uncertainty, dysfunctions that may be significantly compensated for. Thus, many a dyslexic has compensated and overcome almost all of his symptoms: There are dyslexic doctors, dentists, lawyers, engineers, architects, scientists, politicians, and generals.

How could these successful dyslexic adults have become successful if they were still reading two or more years behind their peers? How could they have succeeded if they failed to understand the meaning of letters and words?

What do we call dyslexics who have compensated for their reading deficiencies and now read normally or even above normal levels? Are they suddenly not dyslexic once their reading scores cross the "magic" two-year limit? If indeed their reading scores worsen again, and their scores fall two grades below those of their peers, do they suddenly become dyslexic again?

Of course not! The whole concept of diagnosing dyslexia on the basis of reading scores is completely nonsensical. And yet, many experts fervently believe in this nonsense.

Unfortunately, I did too. However, scientific reality eventually prevailed and I came to recognize that some dyslexics read better than they spell, write, or recall math and directional sequences. Others spell better than they read, while still others can do math better than they read, spell, or write. In short, the symptoms in dyslexia vary in intensity from one dyslexic to another. And the combinations of symptoms may vary significantly from one dyslexic to the next, too.

From this insight I recognized that my daughters Laura and Joy were dyslexic despite their normal and even superior reading abilities. Also as a result of this insight I was fortunately able to treat them effectively. I also came to recognize that dyslexics need not have normal or superior IQs to be dyslexic, and that IQ and dyslexia have nothing to do with one another, contrary to another misconception held by many dyslexia "experts."

Moreover, I eventually realized that dyslexia need not occur in "pure" form. I discovered that mentally retarded, cerebral-palsied, and deaf patients may also be dyslexic, in such cases the retardation, cerebral palsy, or deafness is due to damage to one part of the brain or nervous system while the dyslexia is due to damage to or dysfunction of the inner-ear system.

In a similar fashion I discovered that dyslexia need not occur before or during birth. It may be acquired as a result of any infectious, toxic, trauma, or degenerative process's impairing inner-ear functioning. I realized that ear infections, allergies, toxins, chemicals, head traumas, and whiplash injuries, as well as multiple sclerosis, may impair inner-ear functioning and result in *acquired* dyslexialike functioning. Inasmuch as the medications I used to treat "pure" dyslexics improved inner-ear dysfunction, I came to realize that these very same medications also improve the same symptoms in mixed and acquired dyslexic disorders. In recognizing that most mentally retarded individuals also have a hidden impairment of the inner-ear system (cerebellum), treating their dyslexia has resulted in the first significant improvement in the overall functioning of the retarded.

Dyslexia "experts" have always thought in terms of black and white. You were either cerebral-palsied or dyslexic; you were either deaf or dyslexic. Not true! Many individuals are deaf because of impairment or injury to the nerve that conducts sound impulses to the brain. However, the inner-ear nerve runs alongside this hearing nerve. And, not infrequently, damage to the hearing nerve results in an overlooked damage to the inner-ear nerve.

Invariably all the learning difficulties of the deaf have been arbitrarily attributed to either the deafness or the emotional disturbances resulting from the deafness. No one thought that the learning difficulties in deafness may also be due to the presence of a coexisting but hidden dyslexia. On the basis of this knowledge I have been able to help a number of deaf individuals with their academic difficulties. Moreover, the same medication that helps their academic symptoms often minimizes some of the deafness by improving their auditory sequencing abilities. Even "pure" dyslexics with auditory sequencing difficulties experience a significant improvement in their hearing or auditory memory for phonics and related patterns once they respond favorably to medication.

Without exception, all the learning and motor difficulties in the retarded have been blamed on the impairment resulting in the retardation despite the obvious presence of dyslexic symptoms. And on and on these oversights go. I thought the same way until my patients, their symptoms, and my desire to help them forced me to change my mind.

Most clinicians see four times as many male dyslexics as female dyslexics. Naturally it was assumed that dyslexia is a sex-linked hereditary disorder occurring four times more frequently in males. Wrong again! As stated earlier, I personally screened over 1,500 kindergarten children at a Queens, New York, school district, utilizing my 3-D Optical Scanner. The results of this study indicate that the incidence of male dyslexics equals that of female dyslexics. Male dyslexics are merely referred to clinicians four times more often than female dyslexics. And experts confused the male-female *referral* ratio with the true male-female *incidence* ratio. This is because boys with dyslexia become more frustrated, feel dumber, and act out their frustrations more than girls. Hence they are referred to experts four times more frequently.*

Many an expert still believes that left-handedness and dyslexia are somehow related. My studies have tended to disprove this relationship.

Before completing this highly condensed summary of my research efforts and their outcome, I would like to mention how one of my initial oversights led to a new means of helping dyslexics physiologically while simultaneously enabling me to improve significantly the reliability of my blurring-speed instrument.

After years of using my 3-D Optical Scanner, and after obtaining significant numbers of atypical and paradoxical correlations of poor reading ability and high blurring speeds, I one day discovered that dyslexics have more than one blurring speed. They have the same blurring speed as nondyslexics do—a *sequential blurring speed,* in which a whole sequence is seen as a panorama and the whole blurs out at once. However, they also have another blurring speed, which I called the *single-targeting* blurring speed. This second tracking mechanism is a compensatory one and takes over when the first—the reflexive, sequential-tracking mechanism—is impaired.

For years I assumed, and even demonstrated, that dyslexics can compensate for their blurring speeds independently of their reading scores.

---

*In a personal communication and research paper, Kohen-Raz noted the following seemingly paradoxical findings.

- Normal-reading young girls demonstrate significantly better balance functions than corresponding boys.

- Poor-reading girls demonstrate significantly poorer balance functions than corresponding boys.

To explain this data, I reasoned as follows:

Inasmuch as normal-reading girls have better balance and, thus, inner-ear functioning, they may be expected to better compensate physiologically for any given dyslexic disorder—thus contributing to the 4:1 male/female referral ratio.

- Inasmuch as young normal girls have better developed inner-ear functioning relative to boys, girls may require greater degrees of inner-ear impairment in order to result in impaired reading scores—thus accounting for the presence of poorer balance functioning in reading-score–deficient girls vs. boys.

[R. Kohen-Raz, Ph.D., "Developmental Patterns of Static Balance Ability and Their Relation to Cognitive School Readiness" *Pediatrics,* Vol. 46, No. 2 (August 1970), pp 276–284.]

Thus, for example, eye-training exercises performed by optometrists and me frequently resulted in increased tracking capacity and blurring speeds, with and without a corresponding improvement in reading and related functioning. I knew that compensatory tracking mechanisms were responsible for the atypical and confusing data I obtained, as well as the fact that the blurring-speed methodology was only 80 to 85 percent effective diagnostically rather than 100 percent effective. However, I could not specifically identify or understand the quality of the elusive compensatory tracking mechanism responsible for the seemingly impossible data I had frequently obtained.

This elusive tracking mechanism called single-targeting evaded my grasp for years until I discovered it by accident one day when an adult dyslexic patient suddenly asked me: "Which blurring speed do you want?" Needless to say, I was waiting for several years for someone to give me a clue as to the tracking mechanism responsible for explaining a host of atypical and seemingly paradoxical findings. Upon detailed questioning, this patient told me that she could either follow all the elephants and see them at once until they blurred out, or she could just follow one or two at a time until they blurred out. The first blurring speed was her sequential blurring speed. The second blurring speed was her compensatory single-targeting blurring speed.

The single-targeting mechanism explained why approximately 15 to 20 percent of dyslexics appeared to have normal blurring speeds and why a few dyslexics even reported above-normal blurring speeds. These dyslexics obviously had developed a compensatory tracking mechanism, but the mechanism remained unclear until it was explained to me in great detail by this adult patient.

The concept of a single-targeting tracking mechanism also explained another puzzling finding. I had always assumed that the blurring speed would equal the recognition speed. Let me explain what I mean. If a moving visual sequence is speeded up to the blurring speed, one cannot identify the moving sequence: It looks like a blurred streak. If this blurred streak is slowed up ever so slightly, it can then be identified or recognized. This I called the recognition speed. Thus, during testing, one can speed targets up to the blurring speed, down to the recognition speed, and back up again. This procedure can clearly define the blurring speed with a significant degree of accuracy.

Repeated studies demonstrated that there was no significant difference between the blurring-speed and recognition-speed end points.

I had always thought that the recognition speed would be easier to use to test very young children. One could thus avoid explaining to them exactly what blurring is and means. All I had to ask a young child was: "Tell me what you see as soon as you see it." However, upon further study I came to realize that the blurring speed did *not* always equal the recognition speed, as I had predicted. Thus, for example, the research group who attempted to duplicate my blurring-speed findings could not find a correlation between blurring speeds and reading scores. In retrospect the difficulties were easy to explain: They apparently used recognition speed rather than blurring speed as the end point.

At the time, however, it made perfect theoretical sense to do so, although the results they obtained were most confusing and defied any sensible explanation for many years. They found too many severely impaired readers reporting normal and even above-normal blurring speeds. And the overall dyslexic blurring speeds they obtained were significantly higher than those I obtained myself.

Only later was it easy to understand and explain the research group's findings. In the beginning it was pure torture and frustration. I was extremely disappointed and dejected. I knew my blurring-speed method had to work, for I had been using it for several years. How were the contradictory results to be explained?

Single-targeting, of course, explained it all. If one asks a dyslexic individual, or even a normal individual, to recognize whatever they are seeing, they can identify a single-targeted elephant as easily as they can identify a sequentially targeted elephant sequence. Initially they were not asked to distinguish between the two. All they were asked was: "Tell me what you see as soon as you see it." And indeed they did. They reported seeing elephants. I naturally assumed that dyslexics and nondyslexics saw the elephants in exactly the same way.

They did not!

Dyslexics most frequently were viewing only one elephant at a time, whereas normals were viewing a sequence of eight elephants. Who could have predicted that dyslexics had more than one blurring speed and, as a result of a hidden procedural inconsistency, that dyslexic blurring speeds going up did not equal their recognition or blurring speeds going down? Who could have foreseen that this procedural error inadvertently resulted in our measuring sequential blurring speeds going up and compensatory single-targeting or recognition speeds coming down?

Thus, for example, when *I* tested dyslexics for blurring speeds, I asked them: "Tell me as soon as the elephants initially begin to blur." I then obtained a majority of sequential blurring speeds interspersed with some single-targeting blurring speeds, the latter accounting for the unusual and seemingly paradoxical blurring-speed data previously defying explanation.

When another research group tested dyslexics, they asked: "Tell me as soon as you can see or recognize the elephants." In other words they began testing children who were watching a complete blur and then slowed down the speed of the moving targets until something could be identified. This research team obtained a vast majority of single-targeting blurring or recognition speeds with only a taint of sequential blurring or recognition speeds.

Inasmuch as there exists a 2:1 to 4:1 difference between dyslexic single-targeting blurring speeds and sequential blurring speeds, and in view of the fact that a majority of dyslexics learn to single-target, almost all of the confusing and contradictory results obtained between my data and the independently obtained data were suddenly explained. By recognizing the distinction between the diagnostic sequential-target blurring speed and the much higher compensatory single-target speed, and by correcting the procedural errors in the blurring-speed techniques, the 3-D Optical Scanner jumped from 80 percent effective to over 95 percent effective in diagnostic accuracy. Moreover, the gap between dyslexic's sequential blurring speeds and normal blurring speeds widened from 2:1 to 4:1, making it significantly easier to separate dyslexics from nondyslexic groupings. In addition, the realization that dyslexics may have poor, normal, or superior reading scores helped explain the remaining inconsistencies in attempting to correlate blurring speeds with low reading scores.

Needless to say, if the reading scores of dyslexics varied from one extreme to another, then there could not be a significant correlation between low blurring speeds and low reading scores. After all, my instrument was designed to diagnose dyslexia, not reading scores.

By analogy, the surprising finding that dyslexic blurring speeds going up did not equal dyslexic blurring (recognition) speeds coming down mirrored the fallacy of the assumption that the process whereby cortically impaired adults lost their reading ability equaled the process in which dyslexic children failed to acquire normal reading ability. Having recognized that single-targeting was a compensatory tracking mechanism that may be improved by tracking exercises, I came to realize that the dyslexic who follows one elephant at a time is merely emulating what most dyslexics do when they initially begin reading: They use their finger for a pointer to track one word at a time. In other words single targeting is a learned mechanism by which the brain develops a "mental finger" that guides the eye in time and space so that it can follow a target that is rapidly moving across one's visual field. Without this "mental finger" as a guide, dyslexics' eyes would be lost in space and so would the visual targets.

The discovery of the single-targeting mechanism not only explained a whole series of facts and dramatically improved the diagnostic and screening accuracy of the blurring-speed method and instrument, it underscored a very, very important fact in science: You can spend a tremendous amount of time with data and come to know that something is missing without being able to find it. In such a case, statistical results may appear to invalidate your findings. However, if one really understands the subject matter and the data qualitatively, then one knows how to evaluate and interpret the significance of the statistics. Negative statistics, of course, are important. But simply because they appear to negate one's perceptions does not necessarily mean that these observations are incorrect. It may mean that there is a procedural error somewhere that has thus far been unidentified.

Fortunately, I had been working and living with dyslexics for years and years and I felt I understood their clinical symptoms. I had seen their improvements. I *knew* they had a tracking defect. Just read through the majority of my case histories: All of them, or almost all of them, reported tracking difficulties. Thus, I knew that somehow, somewhere, I would find the missing tracking mechanism needed to explain *all* the findings— the majority as well as the minority, the typical as well as the atypical, the expected as well as the unexpected. I was waiting several years for a clue I could recognize, and consequently was already attuned to my patient's question, "Which blurring speed do you want?" when it was finally asked.

We naturally assume that everyone sees the same way. This is most certainly not true. Single-targeting dyslexics cannot believe that nondyslexics see a whole elephant sequence in an effortless panorama. Parents are astonished, even horrified, when they witness their children reporting seeing only one out of eight elephants.

My 3-D Optical Scanner is a very simple test. But the variations it uncovers could not have been detected had I not performed over 20,000 tests myself. The detection of each and every individual tracking variation and compensation led to ever-expanding insights into inner-ear dysfunctions, dyslexia, and the fascinating ways the brain adapts.

Moreover, the blurring-speed tests revealed a number of findings that were helpful in developing new and useful educational procedures. For example, the blurring speeds of big, black, and colored words or designs were significantly higher than the corresponding blurring speeds for small, light gray, uncolored print spaced closer together. Put another way, reflex eye mechanisms were better able to fixate on, track, and process big, dark, or brightly colored, more widely spaced print, suggesting that printed material and books be appropriately designed for dyslexics, especially those whose tracking mechanisms remain significantly deficient.

By recognizing that young dyslexics have significant tracking difficulties while their eyesight or visual acuity is often within normal limits, I developed an instrument capable of projecting letters and words on a single spot so that the need for eye tracking was minimized. Hence, if the letters and words in a sentence are projected one at a time on a given spot, word recognition and reading can be taught with minimal visual scrambling. Of course, this "reading" process should be carried out simultaneously with attempts to improve the eye-tracking mechanism via repetition and video games.

In addition, the ability to measure auditory and tactile sequencing by means of the 3-D Auditory and Tactile scanners has led to insights into how "open" these respective channels are for teaching purposes. Moreover it is anticipated that auditory and tactile conditioning or training will enable these channels to function better, just as visual tracking exercises result in increased visual tracking capacity and blurring speeds.

This brief history of my research efforts will enable you to develop a better perspective on the methods and means leading me to solve the dyslexic riddle. This solution would never have occurred had I overlooked or denied the significance of data I initially could not account for or explain.

9

The Symptoms and Mechanisms Defining Dyslexia

Introduction

IN MANY WAYS THIS CHAPTER IS THE MOST IMPORTANT AND insightful one in the book, albeit the most detailed and complex. However, I feel its content is well worth your effort. The following truly describes and represents the dyslexic symptomatic core and span, as well as the variations typifying this scientifically misunderstood and elusive disorder.

The analysis of more than 10,000 dyslexia cases during the last twenty years has led me to view this fascinating yet devastating condition as an inner-ear dysfunction affecting any or all of thirteen major categories of functioning:

- (1) Reading
- (2) Writing
- (3) Spelling
- (4) Mathematics
- (5) Memory
- (6) Direction
- (7) Time
- (8) Speech
- (9) Grammar
- (10) Hyperactivity, overactivity, and impulsiveness

(11)   Concentration and distractibility
(12)   Phobias and related mental and behavioral disorders
(13)   Balance and coordination.

In this chapter I describe in great detail the various inner-ear–related dysfunctioning versus compensatory mechanisms and symptoms characteristic of this sample of 10,000 dyslexics. This is the largest such sample ever recorded and analyzed. The recorded symptoms and mechanisms did not readily materialize or fall into place easily. Quite the contrary:

- Each and every symptom was painstakingly collected and studied for years before its true meaning and significance were recognized.
- Each and every symptom was analyzed to determine the underlying mechanisms responsible for its creation.
- Each and every symptom was eventually statistically analyzed so that its relative incidence and frequency was determined in large dyslexic samples.
- Each and every exceptional, atypical, and unexpected finding was studied and analyzed with the same, perhaps more, interest and determination given to the symptoms occurring most typically and frequently.

Oddly enough, reading, writing, spelling, and other scores were not at all helpful in correlating and defining the nature and symptoms characterizing the dyslexic panorama. Indeed, the numbers and scores typifying the traditional dyslexic and learning disability research approaches were most often confusing and misleading. Thus, for example, dyslexia was most commonly viewed and defined as a *severe* reading disorder in which an otherwise completely "normal" individual must be two or more years behind equally matched peers, i.e., equally matched for IQ, socioeconomic, psychological, and educational factors. Is this matching process really possible?

This definition was eventually discovered by me to be completely wrong, even foolish. Bright, exceptionally gifted children were found to have normal reading scores but poor, "typically" dyslexic writing and spelling patterns. According to the prevailing definition of dyslexia, these children were certainly not viewed as dyslexic. Instead they were mistakenly judged to have only average intelligence. These gifted, hardworking children were frequently termed "lazy" and/or "academically indifferent."

Quite a distortion! But how else are traditionally biased experts expected to think? We are unwittingly taught or expected to reason as follows: If the clinical facts do not fit the theory, then the facts are wrong!

To make matters worse, most frequently the gifted dyslexic children who managed to read on or close to grade level are refused help. Once again the traditionally molded experts reasoned: Why do they need help? Are they not reading on grade level, and sometimes even above? None of the educational or psychological testers asked these children the questions necessary to determine whether or not they were experiencing difficulties within their reading processes, difficulties such as memory instability for letters, words, sentences, and paragraphs; reversals; and tracking problems. In other words experts invariably equated normal reading scores with normal reading processes. Unfortunately this equation was incomplete and often completely wrong.

Why didn't these experts reason as follows: If a gifted, hardworking child has only a normal reading score, what dysfunctioning mechanisms are preventing his scores from becoming as superior as is his IQ and effort? Why is this gifted child writing and spelling as if he is dyslexic?

All too often, if the clinical reality did not fit the ingrained theory, then the clinical reality was unwittingly denied:

- The child's IQ was not really high but merely average.
- The child was not really as hardworking as his family believed.
- The child was either not asked the specific questions needed to elicit the typical dyslexic reading symptoms, or these obvious or readily apparent symptoms were denied and were attributed to nondyslexic factors, such as developmental lag and immaturity.
- The typical dyslexic writing, spelling, etc., qualities were denied their proper significance and accordingly sidestepped.

Before continuing, I would like to present you with a typical dyslexic case examined by me on October 5, 1983. The patient's mother writes:

I had been to the public schools many times to seek help for David's reading and spelling problems, but to no avail. All his teachers, along with the reading teacher, told me was that he was just "an average kid who was reading on grade level" and why was I pushing him so hard? They said I would only frustrate David if I pushed too hard. I knew David was bright. They didn't. My "average kid" turned out to have an IQ of over 130 with a learning disability. He's now in a school for gifted children, is being helped by a [learning-disabilities] teacher, and is finally feeling good about himself.

Cases similar to this one—similar to those of my daughters Laura and Joy—eventually forced me to abandon completely the traditional views and definitions of dyslexia.

Dyslexia is not just a severe reading disorder with characteristics of reversals. In fact, the reading scores of dyslexics may be normal and even superior, and reversals may or may not be present. I came to realize that dyslexics frequently compensate for symptoms revealed by traditional testing but are nonetheless still dyslexic. Thus, they may compensate for some reading mechanisms and not others, while the writing and spelling symptoms may remain, appearing as bad as ever. I also came to realize that although most dyslexics are referred to clinicians for severe reading difficulties, there are many dyslexics who compensate for their reading. However, they may experience great frustration with their writing, spelling, math, or concentration.

After years of painstaking clinical and theoretical effort, I reached the simple understanding that dyslexics, not experts, truly define the dyslexic disorder. In other words the patients and the quality of their revealed symptoms are diagnostically correct: If their facts do not fit our established and ingrained theories, then our theories are wrong and must be changed. As a result of major theoretical changes, I arrived at the rather simple, obvious conclusion that any given dyslexic may experience the most frustration with *any one* or *any combination* of categories (1) to (13) listed on pages 108–109.

What happens when a common virus affects five members of a family? Do all members exhibit the same symptoms with uniform intensity? Obviously not! Most frequently each member will evidence some symptoms of the virus, but the leading symptom may be different and the symptom's relative intensity may vary from one extreme to another. In fact, one member of such a family may even feel "almost" well and thus escape clinical detection altogether. The same is true for many a dyslexic.

I will now present you with the thirteen major categories and symptoms categorizing and defining dyslexia.

Reading

The vast majority of young dyslexics referred for clinical evaluation demonstrate a visual and/or phonetic memory instability for letters and words. Hence they repeatedly attempt to recall the shapes and sounds of letter and word configurations only to forget them rapidly. To compensate, many a youngster will initially resort to guessing and even recalling stories by sheer rote, so that often their reading difficulty is not diagnosed until several years later.

Directional disturbances are also frequently present, compounding memory instability by triggering the confusion of such letters and words as *b* with *d, was* with *saw, on* with *no,* and *god* with *dog.*

Fixation and eye-tracking difficulties are invariably present during the dyslexic reading process, and the eye loses its place as it scans letters, words, and sentences. Accordingly letters, words, and sentences are skipped over, resulting in poor concentration and comprehension difficulties. Thus a child cannot understand what he is reading, as the sequence of what his eyes are looking at is significantly scrambled.

As a result of this inner-ear–related tracking difficulty, small words are frequently skipped over completely, resulting in the seemingly paradoxical situation in which small words are harder to recognize than larger words. (Larger words are easier to target and thus recall.) Moreover, letters, syllables, and word parts are frequently skipped over, resulting in the mistaking of *p* for *o* or *l*, *t* for *i*, *read* for *red*, *us* for *bus*, etc. At times, segments of one word are inadvertently carried by the eye to more distant word segments, resulting in fusion or condensation errors; the dyslexic may see *the cat* or *good boy* and read *that* and *go by*. By reviewing the possible errors and mechanisms resulting when a dyslexic reads the sentence "The cat jumped over the moon," you will get a clear understanding of how to analyze the mistakes and better understand the mechanisms responsible for these mistakes.

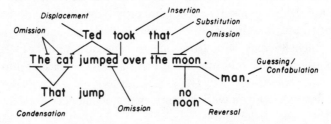

The "typical" dyslexic errors and mechanisms triggered when a reading-disabled sample attempts to read the sentence *The cat jumped over the moon*. By means of an error analysis and diagram, the mechanisms underlying the dyslexic reading performance are reconstructed: omissions, insertions, displacements, condensations, rotations/reversals/scrambling, substitutions, and guessing/confabulation.

The sequential scrambling or tracking dysfunction characterizing the dyslexic reading process results in the omission or disappearance of letters, words, and even sentences from their proper positions. Often these very segments are *displaced* or carried over to new positions, giving rise to the formation of new letters, words, and sentences. Thus the original visual text or sequence becomes significantly distorted by the underlying scrambling processes.

If, in addition, there exists a similar phonetic or sound-sequencing disturbance that parallels the visual one, then there will be utter chaos and frustration, regardless of the individual's IQ. Phonetic or auditory input blurring, distortions, and reversals characterize the dyslexic reading process as frequently as do the visual symptoms.

Because of the visual and auditory defects in dyslexics, words or sounds may appear blurry or muddled. At times the eye or ear appears stuck or fixed to a word, finding it difficult to let go and proceed, or uncontrollably returning to the same word over and over again in an obsessive-compulsive–like fashion, called perseveration. If the same symptom or mechanism affects mental or thought-processing, it may result in the inability to free one's mind from a thought, concern, or tune, psychiatrically referred to as an emotionally determined obsessive disorder. If the same symptom leads to a compelling need to repeat the same motor task over and over again, then compulsions occur.

Underlying many so-called mental symptoms are physically based dyslexialike mechanisms. (Even dreams are characterized by the same fusion and displacement mechanisms characterizing the dyslexic reading processes.) Inasmuch as the eyes' "guided-missile system" is impaired, it is reasonable to expect it to hit big, dark, colored targets rather than small, light, almost invisible ones. For this very reason magnification of letters and words by lenses as a rule results in reading improvement in dyslexics despite the absence of visual acuity problems.

There is, however, one interesting exception to this rule. If eye perseveration is significantly present, and thus the eye cannot free itself from a given target or word, then the smaller the perseveration target, the more readily the eye will escape it, freeing itself to move on to the task at hand.

Frequently the tracking defect in dyslexia does not become obvious until a child gets into the upper grades, where the reading rate must increase in order to accommodate the greater reading volume, and where the print size correspondingly shrinks to accommodate this larger volume. To compensate for the tracking defect, the reading process must be slowed down, and often a marker is needed to direct the eye's movement in space. In this case, one's finger or marker acts as a pacemaker, slowing down the eye's movement while simultaneously serving as a reference point for the zigzagging eye, thus stabilizing and guiding its ability to fixate and sequentially track the words and sentences in their appropriate places.

If, however, eye perseveration is present, then even a finger or a marker as a compensatory device fails. The eye will then fixate on the finger or marker and will not let go. Letters, words, and sentences will then appear blurry and scrambled and thus difficult to read. To compensate, the *mind* develops a *mental finger* and slowly guides the eye from letter to letter and from word to word, adaptively blocking out all adjacent or peripheral distracting impressions. This process is analogous to a compensatory type of tunnel vision. It was this mechanism that I later termed single-targeting.

Compensatory single-targeting mechanisms are forced to develop when teachers and peers ridicule children who use a finger to read or when the finger cannot be used. Similar compensatory mechanisms were later found to occur during the processing of sequential sounds, touch sensations, and related sensorimotor tasks.

Difficulties with concentration and distractibility also complicate the dyslexic reading process. Obviously poor concentration results in rapid fatigue and boredom, rendering distracting background noises and events "louder." As a result, impaired memory and directional and tracking mechanisms are secondarily intensified, further complicating an already complicated process.

Often dyslexics will belatedly develop evidence of a reading difficulty upon entering high school or college, where the rate, volume, and quantity of facts to be recalled are significantly intensified. Prior compensatory mechanisms or skills may be insufficient at this point, and it suddenly appears as if a new problem has arisen. Most frequently it is not a new problem; it is merely the surfacing of an old, hidden, partially compensated-for dyslexic variation.

High school and college problems are most frequently viewed as emotional in origin, and the affected individuals are frequently termed lazy or disinterested. Few educators and clinicians have the experience and good fortune to recognize fully the scope and variations of the reading processes in compensating or partially compensating dyslexics. Thus they cannot distinguish the quality of the dyslexic reading process from nondyslexic disturbances. Erroneous assumptions and diagnoses are made, resulting in mistreatment.

Low reading scores alone cannot distinguish the origin of the poor reading performance. Poor reading ability may result from improper teaching, psychological factors, true disinterest, nondyslexic medical and neurological difficulties, or dyslexia. Fortunately the quality of the dyslexic reading disturbance clearly separates this disorder from all the others, as detected with my 3-D Optical Scanner.

Dyslexics frequently complain of a host of what appear to be psychosomatic symptoms during reading: headaches, dizziness, nausea, double vision, blurred vision, word and sentence movement, changes in word size, colored or black background streaking, etc.

Significant variations in reading memory characterize the dyslexic reading process. For example, some dyslexics read and recall scientific material more readily than novels. For others the reverse is true. Analysis of countless adult dyslexics has revealed the unexpected fact that the compensatory ease and facility they develop in processing and remembering reading information frequently determines interest rather than the reverse. It is a given fact for *all* individuals that interest results in improved concentration, memory, and thus reading success.

Upon further exploration an additional array of dyslexic reading symptoms materialized: head-tilting; reading up close, from far away, or shifting from close to far; blinking; sensitivity to fluorescent and/or natural light; and postural reading preferences, i.e., sitting up, lying down, or tilted. The attempt to understand and explain each and every symptomatic variation has resulted in a concept of dyslexia that encompasses all the symptoms found, the typical as well as the atypical.

The analysis of the above symptoms led to the insight that some symptoms reflect the presence of disturbed mechanisms, while others indicate the presence of compensatory mechanisms. Therefore headaches, dizziness, nausea, motion sickness, blurred and double vision, and word movement reflect disturbances resulting from impaired focusing, tracking, orientation, and memory mechanisms. On the other hand, blinking, finger-pointing, and head-tilting are adaptive attempts at compensation. Blinking, refocusing, and positional shifting as well as head-tilting all attempt to correct for the blurred, double, moving, and changing visual images. The body's inner "gyroscope" is tilted and out of position, and the above maneuvers reflect adaptive attempts to stabilize and realign this "gyroscope."

Many dyslexics will develop rapid scanning devices whereby their eyes "intuitively" pick up key words and phrases; often they are assumed to be superior readers. In fact, my daughter Laura read this way. As a child she was often retested, for teachers could not believe her reading speed. When I eventually retested Laura and others like her, I realized that the rapid scanning was not often in sequence and that she had an uncanny ability to decipher the whole context of a passage from sequentially scattered and incomplete clues. She could not read word by word by word without using her finger and small print tended to blur out quite rapidly for her.

Another patient of mine read from right to left and from the bottom up. His mind then appropriately reversed and translated the stored content and made sense out of it. He could not track in what we consider the normal left-to-right and top-to-bottom directions. Indeed, many dyslexics can mirror-read and comprehend reversed images better than they can read normally.

With time and effort, many of these dyslexic symptoms and mechanisms may be compensated for, resulting in improved functioning. Most often, improvement is frustratingly slow and requires significant degrees of effort. At other times improvement appears sudden and dramatic. When the improvement is slow, the dyslexic is often mistakenly called a "slow learner"; when fast, he is termed a "late bloomer." My studies, however, have clearly shown that "late blooming" may occur early, i.e., prior to kindergarten or in first grade. Late blooming may even occur as late as junior high school, high school, college, or even graduate school.

A host of descriptive terms have been misused as if they described different diagnostic categories. In fact, a slew of terms merely described different speeds and styles of compensation for one and the same underlying disorder. No wonder experts were unable to distinguish clearly the slow learner from the dyslexic! Most often there was no basic distinction other than the speed at which the dyslexic compensated or the intensity of symptoms defining his or her particular type of dyslexia.

The dyslexic reading process is far from stable. It may, and does, regress. Thus fatigue, dyes, allergies, toxins, metabolic and chemical disorders, mononucleosis, ear infections, and concussions may destabilize a preexisting condition and result in variations that are most often misunderstood and, again, misdiagnosed.

Before completing this lengthy but highly condensed description of the symptoms and mechanisms characterizing the dyslexic reading process, I would like to add a few more *exceptional* reading styles.

Although most dyslexics dread reading aloud, for it highlights their slow, poor reading capacity while distracting and disorganizing their already stressed compensatory mechanisms, other dyslexics can remember or know what they visually see only if they hear themselves say it.

The most fascinating style of all is one told to me by several dyslexic artists. They cannot decipher the meaning of a word by viewing the individual letters. Instead they learn the word's meaning by recalling the shape of the overall configuration, i.e., the highs and lows of the letters constituting the words. This interesting mechanism appears to be similar to a mechanism reported to me by other dyslexics whereby they recognize the meaning of a word only after their eyes traverse the word's outline, a reading form I chose to call ocular [eye] braille. By now the reader must surely know that dyslexia—its mechanisms, its symptoms, and its compensatory style—is far from a simple disorder. Certainly it is too complex a disorder to be defined by reading scores, and too complex a disorder to be understood by the rapid examination of relatively small samples.

Each and every symptom and compensatory mechanism of dyslexia was slowly and painstakingly discovered over a twenty-year period of questioning and requestioning thousands of dyslexics. Slowly but surely, each and every symptomatic exception and compensatory style received as much attention as the symptoms recurring most frequently.

If a theory is correct, it must be wide and dynamic enough to explain *all* the symptoms and variations. To date, no other theory of dyslexia comes close to explaining the vast majority of symptoms and mechanisms described and to be described in this book. No other research effort has come close to finding the various characteristics that constitute the dyslexic reading process and dyslexia. No other theory has described and explained the various specific compensatory mechanisms that tend to diminish and mask the symptoms' intensity, leading some experts to think that dyslexia is merely an outgrown or overcome developmental lag.

Despite significant masking of its surface symptoms, the core of dyslexia remains for life.

Writing

The writing ability of dyslexics is frequently delayed and appears to be dyscoordinated, reflecting the difficulty they have recalling and utilizing learned motor patterns. The shape, spacing, and direction of the written content frequently has a sloppy, "discombobulated," uneven quality; the words tend to drift in space. Concentration and effort are often needed to compensate, whereupon fatigue invariably leads to a reappearance of the same old pattern.

For some dyslexics printing is easier than writing script, whereas the reverse is true for others. Interestingly the artistically gifted can "draw" the writing in a calligraphic style while remaining unable to write normally in a coordinated fashion.

Analysis of the writing errors in dyslexics revealed that when printing was easier, there existed an ability to harness and compensate by writing one letter at a time, thereby sidestepping the continuous rhythmic flow and stream required to produce script. For those dyslexics who had an easier time with script, the timing and flow utilized for cursive writing was helpful. Put another way, the rhythm required to complete script was found to be as helpful to some dyslexics when handwriting as it is to stutterers when singing (i.e., stuttering frequently disappears when singing and reappears when talking).

During the process of writing, letters and words are frequently omitted or displaced to more distant parts of the written passage, a condition that resembles the fusion and displacement errors characterizing the dyslexic reading process. At times letters are inadvertently repeated, again highlighting the repetitive or perseverative tendency attending writing as well as reading.

Despite the existence of dyslexic artists, drawing was found to be difficult for the majority of dyslexics. Drawings of human figures were not infrequently tilted and off balance, and arms appeared disjointed; fingers were impossible to draw for the vast majority, and were avoided by drawing gloves, hiding hands behind torsos, or resorting to stick figures (mistakenly interpreted as a symptom of masturbatory or castration anxiety by psychiatrists and psychologists). The various psychological interpretations used to explain dyslexic drawings were found to be as erroneous as those used to explain all dyslexic symptoms.

The dyscoordinated and imbalanced drawings of dyslexics reflect the inner chaos they experience in integrating sensorimotor signals. When attempting to copy a series of designs (Bender Gestalt figures), dyslexics commonly shifted the paper or their bodies in attempts to find compensatory stable reference points. Copied designs were frequently rotated and angled off their intended spatial positions. Moreover, angles and curves were poorly formed and shaped.

In general the writing and drawing errors of dyslexics are easily explainable if one refers to the "guided missile" concept. Just picture the computer within our inner-ear (cerebellar) system guiding our hands and fingers in space. Any dysfunction within this computer will result in our hands and pens being poorly guided and directed, thereby accounting for the misdirected and dyscoordinated quality of the errors that characterize the dyslexic writing and drawing processes, exceptions aside.

However, the exceptions must and can be accounted for. Not every motor function and reflex is misguided in dyslexia. The writing function is spared for some dyslexics, whereas only one of several writing functions is spared for others, clearly indicating that each specific motor function or task has its own specific wavelength or circuit on or by which it is processed. This is true of sensory functioning as well. Each piece of information entering the brain is processed on its own specific wavelength. Thus, some input functions may be impaired while others function well and still others are viewed as gifted.

Mirror-writing is not unusual for some dyslexics. One of my left-handed patients wrote only in reverse. As a result of the fracturing of his left hand he was forced to write with his right hand. Lo and behold, he wrote normally.

Leonardo da Vinci frequently mirror-wrote. Historians claim he did so to disguise his thoughts. However, he might have been dyslexic, and his mirror-writing capacity might have been carried into adulthood, just as many dyslexics retain the ability to mirror-read.

Spelling

Although some dyslexics are excellent spellers (one patient I examined was a proofreader), the spelling function in dyslexia is characterized by a significant memory instability, visual and/or phonetic. The letter sequences of words are frequently forgotten as rapidly as they are learned. At times visual recall is better than phonetic, whereas some dyslexics spell entirely via phonetics, with minimal or no visual recall.

Not infrequently, parents will claim a child spells well simply because he receives *100*'s on tests. Further exploration may reveal that many of these so-called good spellers forget the words shortly after the exam is over and that their practical spelling ability is poor. Many dyslexics forget what they learned prior to taking tests, and thus obtain poor spelling grades. In both types of dyslexics, there is a short-term memory defect in spelling; it is just shorter for failing spellers than for passing spellers.

Directional disturbances frequently complicate the spelling process. Letters and syllables are often reversed. Some dyslexics spell orally better than they do when writing, and the determining mechanism was investigated. In dyslexics with poor writing or graphic ability, written spelling is further impaired by a host of dyscoordinating and scrambling writing mechanisms. If, on the other hand, speech functioning is intact, oral spelling scores may better reveal the degree of spelling dysfunctioning.

Spelling can be compensated for by many dyslexics, but certainly not by all.

Mathematics

Mathematical dysfunctioning in dyslexia is initially experienced as an uncertain memory for addition and subtraction facts, requiring compensatory finger- or mental counting. Later on, difficulties arise when learning the multiplication tables. The multiplication facts are learned and then rapidly forgotten unless reinforced by almost continuous repetition. It is interesting that some dyslexics experience more disability with certain of the multiplication tables than others. For example, some dyslexics will have difficulty with the 7's table while with others it may be the 8's.

For the majority of dyslexics, learning the multiplication tables is more difficult than acquiring addition and subtraction facts. However, this is not always true: Surprisingly some dyslexics learn the multiplication tables with normal or almost normal rapidity while still using their fingers to do simple addition and subtraction.

These variations in learning addition, subtraction, and multiplication once again highlight the fact that each specific math function and even subfunction is processed by way of its own corresponding circuit; thus simple circuits may be impaired while more complicated processing occurs with natural ease.

Reversal and scrambling errors result in dyslexics misreading, miswriting, and misremembering number sequences. Accordingly there results a host of dyslexic slips previously considered psychologically motivated and thus called Freudian slips.

The process of writing numbers in columns, and then adding or subtracting them results in characteristic errors. The number columns are frequently crooked. Numbers in column one are inadvertently added to numbers in column two and even three as a result of the same eye-tracking difficulty triggering letter-, word-, and sentence-skipping when reading.

By encouraging young dyslexics to utilize graph paper, I have shown them how to write their numbers in aligned spaces, which in turn enables them to add columns more accurately by utilizing the guidelines provided by the paper.

Not infrequently dyslexics will reverse directions when performing arithmetical functions. Thus, for example, they will add columns from left to right rather than the reverse, further complicating their difficulties. Even $+$, $-$, $\times$, and $\div$ signs are occasionally reversed or confused with one another. For instance, instead of adding two numbers, dyslexics will occasionally subtract them, or will divide instead of multiply.

Many high school and college dyslexics encounter difficulties with algebra, geometry, trigonometry, and calculus. Often they fully comprehend the concepts; they just have trouble remembering the equations and theorems needed for problem-solving. On the other hand, many a dyslexic finds concept retention more difficult than factual retention. Others experience difficulty with both. Fortunately some dyslexics are gifted in higher mathematics despite earlier memory difficulties with simple arithmetic.

Some dyslexics have great difficulty visualizing the dimensions and angles in geometry, while others function remarkably well with spatial relationships, even better than nondyslexics.

In many cases compensated dyslexics have little difficulty with math until high school. Unexpectedly they become frustrated with algebra, geometry, trig, or calculus. Such cases are invariably misdiagnosed and termed lazy or indifferent, as are dyslexic high school students who suddenly experience similar frustration at having to read greater volumes faster than ever, or are required to recall escalating numbers of facts with less time to study than they had before.

Some bright adult dyslexics were noted still to have difficulty counting change. Apparently their calculation channels were initially "blurred out" severely and later anxiety resulted in their phobically avoiding situations that would have led to compensation. As a result of this insight, I realized that some dyslexics blurred out the *ability to remember* concepts, just as others readily blurr out the ability to remember nonconceptual details. In other words dyslexic individuals know the meaning of money; they just cannot easily recall the significant operational steps required to use it or make change. The resulting anxiety and embarrassment lead to secondary conceptual difficulties as an outgrowth of a money phobia.

Many dyslexic teachers learned the basics of simple arithmetic only when forced to teach their first-, second-, and third-grade students. It appears that their initial mathematical difficulties were complicated by severe anxiety factors. And, when forced to teach, the anxiety factors were bypassed. Dyslexics start out being physiologically inefficient at performing certain tasks. Anxiety factors complicate these processes despite the fact that the individuals may eventually learn to compensate physiologically. Thus a physiologically caused disorder may continue as a result of secondary anxiety factors, even though the initial disturbance was compensated for.

Memory*

Specific patterns and types of memory instability play a vital role in reading, writing, spelling, and mathematical delays.

*Problems with memory, balance, coordination, and speech functioning may intensify with age in dyslexics. Patients and clinicians frequently fear they are developing Alzheimer's disease, multiple sclerosis, or even brain tumors.

The analysis of dyslexic functions has clearly revealed that memory is not an all-or-nothing function. One can have a poor memory for visual and word recall while having a great memory for phonetics, and one can easily learn addition and subtraction facts while experiencing extreme frustration when attempting to learn and retain the multiplication tables.

Based on this insight, I was forced to recognize that each and every piece of information is processed, stored, and retrieved independently of other memory functions. Each and every dyslexic will therefore be characterized by a unique quality and pattern of memory functioning versus dysfunctioning or instability.

Upon analyzing the memory functions of large samples of dyslexics, certain characteristics occurred and reoccurred. The following *specific* memory functions were typically delayed or impaired: learning or retaining the names of colors, shapes, people's names and/or faces, important dates, even daily events. In addition, sequential memory functioning frequently appears to be delayed among many dyslexics. Many will experience difficulty recalling their addresses, their telephone numbers, and/or the days of the week and the months of the year in order. Although many of these memory problems are matters of storage, there are retrieval problems as well. For example, the majority of dyslexics experience subtle difficulties recalling words they know and wish to use in ordinary speech. Known proper names frequently remain "on the tip of one's tongue" rather than in one's conscious memory bank. Occasionally a successfully treated adult dyslexic with severe reading and spelling difficulties will suddenly read and spell well without further tutoring. This observation indicates the presence of a memory retrieval problem rather than a storage problem. Needless to say, both types of memory problems may coexist, albeit in varying proportions.

At times remembered facts cannot be appropriately erased. Parents frequently tell me: "My child has a fantastic memory. Once he learns something, even if it is wrong, he won't be able to forget and correct it." If a spelling or number sequence is learned improperly, the same error will be made throughout the individual's life. New and correct memory impressions do not lead to the erasing or correcting of facts incorrectly recorded. Instead, retained misimpressions continue to conflict with newly acquired accurate impressions, resulting in doubt and uncertainty. Dyslexic physicians frequently display the ability to spell recently learned medical terms accurately, whereas their spelling of simple words remains poor.

In many ways a physiological failure to erase memory impressions appears to be similar to the perseveration mechanisms by which the eye becomes stuck to a word, the pen to a letter, the mind to a thought or an action. Even need and desire may be insufficient to neutralize these perseverative mechanisms affecting the eye, the mind, memory functions, and motor tasks.

Specific patterns of memory function and dysfunction vary not only from dyslexic to dyslexic but from time to time, depending upon a host of compensatory and decompensatory circumstances, such as fatigue, infection, and trauma.

Directions

Orientation and directional or spatial difficulties characterize dyslexic functioning, resulting in reversal and scrambling errors affecting reading, writing, spelling, math, memory, and speech. Underlying the directional disturbances is an impairment of the inner ear's compass. Thus dyslexics have difficulty instinctively knowing right and left and at times front and back, up and down, east and west, north and south, etc. With time and learning, this disturbance may be compensated for. Dyslexics often utilize their thinking brains to reason out right and left. For example, a child will know that he writes with his right hand. As a result, when asked to turn right, he'll squeeze his writing hand, recall that his writing hand is his right hand, and in that way know which direction is right.

One of my patients had a wart on his left hand and used it as a means of determining which direction was left. Following the surgical removal of this wart, he once again became bewildered about directions and required another compensatory device. Some dyslexics become easily confused about where they're going and how to get there, even if they have repeated the sequence a number of times before. Occasionally a bright adult dyslexic will tell me that he gets lost each time he goes home. In fact, some patients refuse to move once they have learned to travel to and from their homes. Moreover they will not venture to or from home via a new route.

By contrast, other dyslexics will overcompensate and develop especially keen directional skills. They just seem to know where they are going, even in new places. Ironically some of these "intuitive navigators" remain uncertain about right and left.

The analysis of countless errors and disturbances eventually led me to recognize that many fears of getting lost or going to new places reflect disturbances in directional rather than psychological functioning. In time I realized that many children who frequently get lost, and those who fear to stray and wander, have one and the same difficulty—an inner-ear compass dysfunction.

Time

The inner ear is a pacemaker imparting timing and rhythm to various motor skills. Accordingly a dysfunctioning inner-ear system may result in difficulty or delay in sensing time, as well as difficulty in learning to tell time.

Compensatory and overcompensatory processing may result in "gifted" timing mechanisms whereby dyslexics are able intuitively to measure time spans down to split seconds. Still, they may have difficulties reading an ordinary watch. The difficulties in reading time are manifold:

- Difficulty recalling number representation
- Difficulty recalling hand representation, i.e., which hands tell minutes and hours
- Directional disturbances such as clockwise and counterclockwise, before and after
- Difficulty seeing the numbers clearly, i.e., blurred vision
- Eye-tracking disturbances resulting in skipping and misreading the clock's numbers.

Although digital watches have been lifesavers for many dyslexics, they have presented difficulties for some. Thus *7:15* may easily be misread as *7:51* or any reversal combination thereof.

Speech

Speech disturbances of varying intensity and quality characterize a majority of dyslexics. While some speech difficulties are readily apparent, the vast majority are subtle and are elicited only upon careful questioning.

Many a future dyslexic will have been a late talker, while others will exhibit a variety of articulation or slurring speech errors requiring speech therapy.

Episodic stuttering was found to taint dyslexic samples periodically, suggesting that there is a relationship between stuttering, dyslexia, and inner-ear dysfunction. Later studies of mine clearly verified this relationship.

As stated earlier, the inner ear imparts timing and rhythm to motor tasks, speech included. As a result of a disturbance in rhythmic activity, speech functions may become dysrhythmic, resulting in starting, stopping, and sequential rhythmic errors.

The concept that rhythm is impaired in stuttering is supported by an interesting observation: Stuttering frequently disappears when individuals sing. Some researchers even notice improvement in stuttering when a metronome is placed next to the ear; the former acts as a rhythmic pacemaker. If rhythmic activity helps compensate for stuttering, then might we not further assume that a disturbance in rhythm underlies stuttering?

Starting and stopping speech activity in stuttering was found to be complicated by another factor already described—perseveration. In other words a motor speech pattern becomes stuck and interferes with the normal speech flow. Not infrequently stuttering may also be triggered by difficulty pronouncing or recalling a word or thought. The resulting hesitation will invariably affect speech rhythms, especially if preexisting disturbances are already present.

The most common and subtle disturbances found among dyslexics, often leading many to become shy and avoid unnecessary speaking, are input and output speech lags. In the presence of a drifting sound input, many dyslexics will hear the sound and not know its meaning until several seconds or even several minutes later. If the sound sequence coming into the brain drifts, it will take the thinking brain several seconds or several minutes to compensate for the disturbance, and the patients will frequently ask "What?" This reflex response allows the patient time to compensate for this drifting input and eventually know what was said.

If the motor speech responses drift, or if there are impaired word memory or concentration mechanisms, then there will be a lag between the intention to say something and the actual motor speech response. Memory disturbances for word and thought recall may so complicate the spontaneous speech flow that many dyslexics develop "loose," rambling, and disjointed speaking styles, and are naturally viewed as scatterbrained. This dyslexic speech style must be clinically differentiated by a doctor from more serious neurological and psychological disturbances affecting the speech process, such as those that underlie the loose, rambling speech of psychotic patients or aphasic patients.

Directional disturbances frequently affect speech-processing and result in word and even thought reversals. For this reason dyslexics are prone to slips of the tongue, saying words out of sequence, or reversal of directions such as up and down.

Concentration and distractibility disturbances may further complicate all of the above speech disturbances and mistakenly give the impression of a hearing loss. Hearing tests are recommended in these circumstances.

The inability to inhibit or block out extraneous background noises or speech patterns while listening to someone nearby or in the foreground may result in severe confusion for some dyslexics. The background contaminates and scrambles the foreground sound sequence and results in an overall sound blurring. This type of situation is frequently present in crowds and restaurants and was found to result in crowd and restaurant phobias.

Grammar

Many dyslexics experience great difficulty in understanding and/or utilizing simple grammatical forms. This disturbance affects written expression much more commonly than verbal expression. When grammatical dysfunction is present, writing and/or speech becomes rambling and run-on in quality and form.

Complex grammar is also affected by the dyslexic disorder. However, this disturbance is more difficult to analyze, for the teaching and learning of grammar varies significantly with educational instruction.

By contrast, every eight-, nine-, or ten-year-old child should know simple grammar, regardless of prior teaching methods.

Hyperactivity, Overactivity, and Impulsiveness

The body's motor and energy levels are frequently improperly fine-tuned by the inner ear in dyslexia. There result hyperactive, overactive—even hypoactive, or decreased activity—levels, as well as fluctuations between these different states.

Dyslexic children may initially show abnormal activity levels at an early age, even from birth. Some mothers have even reported feeling hyperactive fetal activity, clearly suggesting that hyperactive or motor racing states may occur prior to birth.

Hyperactivity is frequently distinguished by its onset. When this symptom occurs in the young or during the preschool years, it is frequently referred to as *developmental* in origin. If this hyperactive, overactive, or restless abnormal motor activity first appears in conjunction with school activity, it may be referred to as *acquired*.

Developmental activity forms are frequently viewed as being of physiological origin, whereas the acquired forms are thought to be of psychological origin. However, my studies clearly show that the developmental and acquired forms may both be of physiological origin, although the acquired form is frequently milder in nature and thus requires the frustration and anxiety of school to trigger it so that it becomes belatedly recognizable. Moreover, the analysis of the so-called developmental and acquired activity states reveals the presence of still another hidden dyslexic mechanism: the inability of an impaired inner-ear system to control, regulate, or dampen anxiety buildup. Hence, a dysfunction within this anxiety-regulation mechanism may result in greater degrees of frustration in so-called developmental than in acquired activity states. Thus abnormal activity levels become more apparent earlier in the developmental state than in the acquired state.

My studies further demonstrate that severe hyperactivity is relatively uncommon in dyslexia. These wild states of "runaway" activity or perpetual-motion activity are most commonly observed in brain-injured children and adults. In contrast, mild degrees of hyperactivity and still milder forms of restless, fidgety, overenergetic activity, all of which I call overactivity, are most frequently observed in dyslexics.

High-activity motor levels or energy levels are frequently associated with a poor or low frustration tolerance and result in impulsive, poorly thought-out behavioral and verbal discharges, such as cursing, temper outbursts, stealing, and truancy. The need to discharge frustration and anxiety rapidly frequently leads to such negative defensive activities as alcoholism, drug abuse, and a series of avoidance or phobic mechanisms: cutting school, avoiding work, etc.

Overactivity is frequently associated with the increased stress and frustration of school activities, and was termed acquired to describe this correlation. My research indicates that the added pressure of school does not invariably cause the abnormal regulation of activity (overactivity); it merely triggers and brings to the surface a previously hidden and compensated-for activity disorder. I therefore came to view "mild" hyperactivity, overactivity, and hypoactivity as mere variations on a common theme. As stated earlier, most often the distinction between developmental and acquired activity dysfunctions was found to be inaccurate and denoted the degree of disturbance rather than a separate causative origin.

There are several reasons justifying my view of hyperactivity, over-activity, and hypoactivity as merely degrees of the same disturbance:

- Frequently one state spontaneously slides into another and even back again.
- Medications helpful for hyperactive states similarly benefit overactive and even hypoactive states.
- These very same medications are helpful regardless of whether the abnormal activity is labeled developmental or acquired.
- All three states appear to be similarly compensated for with time.

One will often read that hyperactivity or overactivity disappear by puberty and that medications are no longer needed or helpful afterward. Although this assumption is true for some dyslexic individuals, it is by no means valid for all. Many hyperactive dyslexic children will act out their frustrations and develop into explosive, impulsive, drifting, anti-social, driven young and older adults. They still require active medical and psychological treatment, even as adults.

Concentration and Distractibility

Disturbances of concentration and distractibility are frequently associated with hyperactive and overactive states. The racing motor commonly in-terferes with normally sustained concentration levels. However, concen-tration may also be independently disturbed, or fragmented, by the drifting sensory input characterizing the dyslexic disorder. Extra concentration effort is then required to compensate, and relative "burn-out" or fatigue rapidly ensues.

In other words, many dyslexics who appear to have short attention spans do not. This illusion is created by the need to expend large amounts of concentration and effort over relatively short periods of time to com-pensate for the drifting input and output channels. Moreover, concentra-tion mechanisms are similarly fine-tuned by the inner-ear system as are motor mechanisms and the sensory channels. Consequently a fine-tuning disturbance will result in drifting concentration levels, or a true short attention span, distractibility, daydreaming, etc.

Normally functioning individuals frequently rest their concentration mechanisms while adequately performing many tasks on a "reflex" level. Dyslexics cannot relax or rest their concentration mechanisms without immediately paying the price: a host of typical dyslexic slips and errors. Dyslexics require sustained concentration mechanisms functioning in high gear to control and compensate for their underlying chaotic sensorimotor channels. There is no rest for the weary dyslexic. He must forever be on guard and remain in an overcontrolled state of high alert.

As a result, some dyslexics compensate and develop superconcentration mechanisms and abilities that resist normal degrees of fatigue and diversion. However, the vast majority are not so fortunate. They are forced to struggle constantly to keep their concentration mechanisms going. Many fail in this attempt and forever complain of feeling sleepy, tired, foggy, in a trance, or blocked.

The relationship between concentration mechanisms and disturbances of inner-ear functioning is significant and fascinating. Not only do concentration efforts and mechanisms help compensate for the typical sensorimotor dyslexic symptoms, these same mechanisms play a major role in minimizing inner-ear-determined motion sickness and related dysfunctions.

Perhaps a few clinical examples will prove helpful here. During special inner-ear testing, called electronystagmography (ENG), the inner ear is stimulated using warm and cool water as well as rotation. These stimuli frequently trigger dizziness, nausea, even vomiting, as well as a reflex pattern of rapid eye movements called nystagmus, especially if individuals are tested with their eyes closed. The above symptoms can be rapidly reversed if:

(1) The subjects are asked to open their eyes
(2) These subjects are asked to calculate or perform tasks requiring concentration
(3) The subjects are asked to fixate and concentrate upon a specific object. This task best and most rapidly serves to eliminate the induced symptoms.

These observations led me to recognize that eye fixation and/or concentration mechanisms inhibit or dampen motion-sickness responses. Similar observations were spontaneously made by dyslexics with motion-sickness tendencies when riding in a car. They are most prone to car sickness when seated in the back. If they sit next to the driver and look out the front window, their car sickness decreases or disappears. Without question they feel best when they are driving, an activity requiring maximum concentration and fixation efforts, and many individuals with motion-sickness tendencies refuse to ride in a car unless they drive.

Psychologists have assumed that the above individuals have a need to control others or to avoid being controlled by others. Not so! They merely wish to avoid motion sickness. They wish to control only their own inner-ear systems!

Upon analysis it became apparent that concentration and eye-fixation mechanisms tend to improve inner-ear functioning and thus result in a decrease in corresponding symptoms. A series of animal experiments demonstrated that visual stimulation results in decreased inner-ear reactivity or sensitivity, corroborating the findings I observed while studying dyslexics.

Repeated observations demonstrated that improved concentration results in a corresponding improvement in sensorimotor functioning. As a result, I began treating dyslexics with concentration-stimulating medications while simultaneously utilizing anti–motion-sickness agents. Accordingly there resulted higher yields and degrees of improvement among my dyslexic patients than when they were treated with only antihistamines. No doubt for similar reasons the astronauts are treated with a combination of anti–motion-sickness and concentration-improving medications.

Distractibility is frequently reported by dyslexics with concentration difficulties despite the fact that this symptom may occur in the presence of intact concentration mechanisms. My research has shown that the inner-ear system acts as a filter separating unwanted background stimuli or noise from important foreground events.

A dysfunctioning inner ear frequently results in impaired filter functioning. In this case visual and/or auditory overloading may occur and give rise to such symptoms as light sensitivity or sound sensitivity. Moreover the visual and/or auditory input may be scrambled by the incompletely separated background and foreground inputs resulting in variations of visual and/or auditory blurring.

Dyslexics with a dysfunctioning filter will often become fearful of crowds, or demophobic. The crowd represents a situation in which there is either too much visual or too much auditory stimulation. The overloading triggers anxiety responses, and the latter in turn triggers avoidance or phobic mechanisms.

Fortunately the same medications that improve concentration mechanisms also result in improvement of the inner ear's filter functioning, thus minimizing or eliminating distractibility. Improvement in concentration by any means will frequently diminish the distractibility resulting from impaired inner-ear functioning. Interesting material presented to dyslexics in a manner that stimulates their concentration invariably results in decreased distractibility and increased inner-ear functioning.

All too often interest and its beneficial effects on learning have been viewed only in psychological or educational terms. My concepts have added a fascinating physiological dimension to the various psychological explanations of motivational learning. Moreover, the use of medications and various physiological conditioning techniques has provided a new medical dimension to the learning-teaching experience.

Before concluding this topic, I would like to leave the reader with a question to ponder: Is it not possible that a series of *sleep* disturbances, such as insomnia, nightmares, and the inability to wake up in the morning; states of fluctuating consciousness, such as dream states, split personality, etc.; and mood disturbances previously thought to be of psychological origin may be in fact also physiologically determined by mechanisms affecting concentration?

Phobias and Related Mental and Behavioral Disorders

Having studied the dyslexic case material presented thus far, it should be obvious to the reader that dyslexics have difficulty processing motion input and are thus prone to motion-related phobias; fears of moving elevators, escalators, cars, planes, trains, buses, carnival rides, crowds, etc. Inasmuch as the scanning mechanisms of dyslexics periodically become fixed or stuck to sensory impressions, thoughts, and motor events, dyslexics are prone to obsessive-compulsive or perseverated symptoms.

Hyperactivity and overactivity states predispose individuals to temper outbursts, drifting and wandering natures, as well as rapid boredom and the inability to stick with tasks, especially when the hyperenergetic states are combined with concentration difficulties. Hypoactivity and low energy levels frequently leave individuals feeling tired, drained, depressed, even introverted. By contrast, racing energy levels predispose or force individuals to exhibit extroverted behavior.

This topic will be developed further in Chapter X, inasmuch as the content is too important and lengthy to remain a mere subgrouping.

Balance and Coordination

As stated, the inner ear regulates all balance and coordination mechanisms; therefore an inner-ear dysfunction will frequently result in some delay or disturbance in balance and coordination mechanisms. As a result of impaired balance and coordination functioning, some dyslexics appear "klutzy" or clumsy, while others—both children and adults—are accident-prone and often bruised and thus appear to be abused. It is interesting that some dyslexics, like Bruce Jenner, through compensation or because they are gifted, become athletes despite poor eye-tracking coordination when reading and impaired writing coordination.

The *majority* of dyslexics are neither extremely "klutzy" nor athletically gifted. Almost all exhibit some dysfunction of balance and coordination, however slight. Even bed-wetting and soiling may result from poorly coordinated motor (involuntary sphincter) control. The so-called anti-depressant medication traditionally used to treat these symptoms was discovered to improve a wide variety of other dyslexic symptoms, es-pecially concentration.

Last, but not least, improperly balanced muscle tone aggravated by the tugging of opposing muscles, may intensify or trigger such symptoms as flat feet; toeing-in and/or -out; knees turning in and/or out; "loose" ligaments, muscles, and joints, as well as "double-jointed" states, buck-ling muscles, and sudden falling; improperly aligned eyes (strabismus); even scoliosis.

Dyslexics have as much difficulty coordinating multiple motor tasks as they have coordinating multiple visual and/or auditory inputs. For example, upon testing, many dyslexics cannot simultaneously talk and perform a repetitive motor task. They are able to do one or the other, but not both. Some dyslexics have difficulty driving a car while listening to the radio or conversation; they cannot concentrate on both tasks at the same time.

Summary

Thirteen major categories of dyslexic functioning as well as their re-spective symptoms and mechanisms have been described. The reader has been provided with both the quality and a qualitative analysis of the wide-ranging symptoms characterizing the dyslexic disorder. Similar symptoms may result from nondyslexic, non–inner-ear mechanisms and causes. Invariably, however, the symptoms' qualities will be distinctly different. Thus dyslexic disorders may be distinguished (by a doctor) from non-dyslexic disorders.

Frequently, psychological and psychiatric stress and crisis, fatigue, concussion states, etc., may trigger the appearance of typical dyslexic symptoms. One usually finds that either a dyslexic or inner-ear disorder already existed and that the trigger merely exaggerated the problem, or an inner-ear disturbance was newly created and therefore the symptoms were newly acquired.

Additional Insights

Before concluding this chapter, I would like to leave the reader with something new to think about.

As mentioned earlier, dyslexics sometimes experience greater difficulty spelling shorter words than they do with longer words, mirroring the greater difficulty some have reading smaller as opposed to larger words. Upon observing the relative ease with which an occasional dyslexic learns to read, write, and spell despite the continued presence of dyslexic reading, writing, and spelling errors—even for simple words—I realized that an important explanatory mechanism was still eluding my grasp. Analysis of the spelling errors characterizing adult dyslexic professionals was needed before the above mechanisms became clear: Dyslexic doctors, dentists, lawyers, and others frequently display more difficulties with smaller words than with the infinitely more complex technical words they learned in graduate school.

One common denominator was found linking these observations: The more difficult words that were found to be easier to recognize, write, and spell were invariably learned when older. I suddenly found an explanation linking all of these seemingly atypical and paradoxical facts:

- In spite of the increasing difficulty needed to process those tasks required for each succeeding grade, with age some dyslexics compensate and thereby find it easier to read, write, and spell.
- If the initial dyslexic misperceptions and conflicting perceptions of the relatively simple reading, writing, and spelling forms are not erased from an individual's memory but instead remain active, imprinted alongside new, correct, compensated learning experiences, then simple letter and word configurations will be remembered incorrectly.
- Newly learned words—more complicated forms—perceived after compensation has occurred do not conflict with previously mislearned forms and are thus more accurately remembered for reading, writing, and spelling.

This seemingly impossible dyslexic learning style, whereby simple words are harder to remember than more complicated words, has led to further investigation and an explanation that has far-reaching importance:

- One cannot glibly tell parents that their children will never learn new languages because of persistent reading, writing, and spelling difficulties with the original "learned" language. Although that prediction is true for the dyslexic majority, there are exceptions, and these exceptions must be dealt with.
- The earlier one treats dyslexics, the less *mislearning* there is, the less time these dyslexic impressions are superimposed upon one another, and the less retained they are.
- The longer dyslexic misfacts are stored and reinforced, the more difficult it is to erase them and the more perseverated they become.
- The same reasoning holds true for the dyslexic mechanisms: The longer they are in force, the more likely they are to remain imprinted forever—perseverated—and consequently the more difficult they are to compensate for academically, medically (even with medications), and psychologically, resulting in irreversible emotional scarring.

The difficulty in erasing early mechanisms and styles of perceptions is consistent with, and can explain a series of, known psychological observations:

- The vivid perceptions of children most frequently dampen with age, a phenomenon similar to what happens with dyslexic symptoms. However, occasionally vivid perception and memory will persist with age, accounting for eidetic or "gifted" visual, auditory, and/or photographic memory functioning in older individuals.
- At times this eidetic style of functioning is a compensatory one for dyslexics, and allows them to compensate for their underlying impairments.
- Childhood neuroses and even psychoses are frequently caused by the retention of early vivid memory or fantasy impressions, which remain unconciously present and active for life, conflicting with newer or more accurately learned impressions. Accordingly the aim of psychotherapy and psychoanalysis is to revive and retrieve these "hidden" false but active impressions and erase them from an individual's memory banks. Conditioning therapies, on the other hand, attempt to bury these perseverated memories still deeper by strengthening newer, more realistic and adaptive memories and mechanisms.

Stated another way, recognition that *early learning* and *early mislearning* may *stick* or *perseverate* as a result of a physiological mechanism affecting memory functioning may help explain:

- The predisposition of some children to neurosis, psychosis, behavior disorders, etc.
- The increased benefits from child psychotherapy versus adult therapy and early learning versus belated learning.

Although perseverated functioning was initially viewed as an unusual and atypical physiological maladaptive mechanism, there exists another completely different explanation.

- If perseverated memory results in the oversticking of memory impressions and difficulty in erasing, might not the absence of normal memory functioning in dyslexics result from rapid erasures and therefore the absence of perseveration?
- Might there not be degrees of perseveration? And might we not have missed this in viewing only extreme rather than normal variations of this sticking mechanism?
- Might not brainwashing or bias be viewed in terms of exaggerated or perseverated memory mechanisms resistant to normal and appropriate erasure?
- Do not bias or perseverated memory patterns coexist with realistic memory patterns, mirroring the manner in which dyslexics simultaneously reverse and misidentify small words more readily than complicated ones? In other words, originally ingrained memory and thought functions may persist, resisting correction or erasure, despite the *coexisting* pressure of *normal*, contradictory memory and thought patterns acquired later.
- Might not acute stress factors, such as that experienced during extreme periods of emotional and physical trauma, trigger perseverationlike memory mechanisms that render forgetting difficult and at times even impossible, resulting in what is psychiatrically referred to as traumatic neurosis, war neurosis, etc.?

Has my attempt to explain a seemingly unusual and statistically atypical event not resulted in insights and speculations never before thought of?

10
Phobias and the Inner Ear

WHO COULD HAVE PREDICTED THAT MY DYSLEXIC RESEARCH would lead me to recognize that the physical basis of a large variety of phobias and related so-called mental disorders was similar to that of dyslexia and its variable symptomatic fallout? Certainly not I!

My psychiatric practice and my studies of dyslexia eventually forced me to draw two unexpected conclusions:

I

The vast variety of phobias seen by psychiatrists did not fit into the traditionally accepted psychoanalytical theories, just as the dyslexic symptoms did not fit into the very same proposed theories. As a result, the understanding, explanation, and response of phobias to psychotherapy and psychoanalysis appeared to be as incomplete as the similar explanations and treatment of dyslexia.

Improvements were noted. Cures were seldom if ever seen. To say the least, crucial scientific explanations and determinants were missing. The traditionally proposed psychological theories that attempted to explain phobias were most incapable of realistically accounting for their shapes, forms, variable intensities, onset, and disappearance, as well as the various combinations of phobias often appearing in any one person.

In other words, given the personality profile and background of any individual, psychiatric theory was unable to explain the specific phobias, or com-

136

binations of phobias, to which he or she might be heir. In fact, there was no way to predict which patients would develop phobias and which would not. Thus traditional theories could not satisfactorily explain why one patient was afraid of cars, another of buses, another of trains, another of planes, another of heights or bridges, another of walking across wide-open areas, another of various combinations of the above; or why still others feared crowds, social events, department stores, food markets, losing control, tunnels, swimming under water (especially with eyes closed) or just plain swimming. . . .

Even the generalized mechanisms assumed responsible for the *universally* occurring phobias escaped comprehensive, meaningful interpretations.

Reluctantly, I was forced to admit that the traditionally accepted and espoused theories of phobias just did not fit or explain the clinical facts of phobic life. Crucial insights were missing. Indeed, there existed a scientific void.

II

Dyslexic children and adults periodically complained of phobias identical to those I attempted to treat and understand in my psychiatric practice. Moreover, many dyslexic patients who were medically treated spontaneously reported significant improvements in their phobias and self-esteem, as well as in their more typical dyslexic symptoms. As the title of this book indicates, the vast majority of my dyslexic patients felt stupid, dumb, and ugly—the very same feelings expressed by my phobic patients in psychiatric treatment.

Was it possible that many phobias were part of the dyslexic disorder? And if so, what were their determining inner-ear mechanisms? Was it possible that my psychiatric, phobic patients were also dyslexic without my knowing it? Could their dyslexia account for their feeling stupid, dumb, and ugly? Might dyslexic or inner-ear mechanisms better account for the shapes, forms, and combinations of phobias than did the traditionally accepted, but significantly incomplete, psychiatric explanations?

Various conditioning therapies and antidepressant medications (or concentration stimulants) appeared to help a significant number of phobic patients. Was it possible that conditioning therapy helped phobics just as eye conditioning and occupational-therapy conditioning helped dyslexics—by improving the functioning of the underlying inner-ear circuitry via "practice-makes-perfect" mechanisms or via compensatory feedback loops?

Do the so-called antidepressants help phobics as they do dyslexics—by improving the strength and force of compensating concentration mechanisms while perhaps simultaneously fine-tuning the mechanisms regulating and controlling anxiety? And do the anti–motion-sickness medications improve the phobias among dyslexics as a result of their improving the underlying inner-ear mechanisms that I now suspected were crucial in determining phobic symptoms in general?

Motion-Related Phobias

These questions triggered answers. And, as the answers seemed to correlate with all the known facts concerning phobias and dyslexia, I became increasingly excited and enthusiastic. Unexpectedly and suddenly the boundaries of dyslexic research expanded beyond belief. I was once again off to a new beginning.

I suddenly knew what elevators, escalators, buses, trains, cars, planes, and walking across wide-open spaces had to do with one another. They were all motion-related!

I knew the inner ear processes the total motion input. And I also knew that the inner ear processes each type and quality of motion via a specific and distinctly different independent circuit, thus accounting for the various forms of motion sickness. For example, one can be carsick and bus-sick without being plane-sick. One can be elevator- and escalator-sick and not be carsick. One can even be prone to circular motion sickness, as on carnival rides, while feeling fine riding in a straight line or moving up and down. In other words, motion sickness is most frequently direction-specific. In some individuals motion sickness and/or dizziness, nausea, and vomiting are triggered by non–motion-related stimuli: visual, auditory, or olfactory signals, even crowds.

From these insights I suddenly knew why phobic individuals are prone to varying patterns and qualities of motion and crowd phobias. Simply stated, the patterns and forms of motion phobias are related to and determined by corresponding patterns of underlying and dysfunctioning inner-ear circuits, which process these motion activities. Moreover, the name of the phobia was found to be relatively irrelevant, merely signifying the *trigger* that provokes or intensifies dysfunctioning inner-ear mechanisms, thus resulting in anxiety, motion sickness, dizziness, and avoidance phenomena, i.e., phobias. Once a specific motion-related situation or circumstance triggers panic, anxiety, dizziness, motion sickness, imbalance, or fear of losing control, this very same situation will be anticipated and avoided in the future.

Since one of the functions of the inner-ear system is to control and regulate motion-related mechanisms, any inner-ear dysfunction and resulting anxiety may predispose some dyslexics to rapid and long-lasting anxiety buildups and anxiety states. Inasmuch as intense, overwhelming, emotionally traumatic anxiety or panic states result in vivid memories and reminders of danger situations, it is only natural that these danger situations will be avoided until the trauma can be emotionally overcome and the memory erased. If, however, this memory, via perseveration, is not readily erased, and if this persisting vivid memory triggers anxiety responses that rapidly escalate, then the memory of the resulting anxiety and panic serves as a second trigger, with both mechanisms and the resulting triggers predisposing an individual to a corresponding phobia.

Non—Motion-Related Phobias

Although the motion-related phobias and one's predisposition to them may now be explained in terms of inner-ear–related mechanisms, the reader may justifiably wonder: Are non–motion-related phobias also triggered via inner-ear mechanisms?

The answer is *yes*! Once I recognized the relationship between the inner ear and motion phobias, it seemed only reasonable to see just how far I could go in analyzing the remaining phobias for possible inner-ear–related determinants and mechanisms.

COMPASS—RELATED PHOBIAS

I had already guessed that dyslexic children who fear getting lost—and dyslexic adults who fear new places and thus avoid traveling—have an underlying compass-related orientation and directional disturbance. Obviously, if one's sense of direction and one's memory for direction are significantly impaired, it is reasonable to avoid straying into new or disorienting situations. Does not the inner ear process compass-related directional, orientational, and memory functions?

SCHOOL PHOBIAS

Upon analysis, most school-phobic children examined by me turned out to be dyslexic. Their school phobia represented an unconscious attempt to avoid the emotionally devastating and humiliating feelings of stupidity triggered by their academic frustration.

According to traditional psychiatric theory, school phobics are over-pampered, overloved, spoiled, "homesick" children, and thus fearful of leaving their parents. Although this theory may hold for a few cases, it is hardly true for the vast majority of school phobics. In the majority of cases the parental concern for their children, and perhaps even overconcern, is secondary to their loving attempts to help their troubled children overcome a frightening and misunderstood "emotional" disorder. In other words psychoanalysts mistakenly viewed concerned parents' attempts to help their children as the cause of the problem. Once again, cause and effect were scientifically found to be reversed.

Ignored by psychiatrists was the obvious fact that most school phobias occur with increasing grade levels, first when the pressure and complexity of schoolwork becomes increasingly difficult. If fears of separating from parents were primarily responsible for this phobia, then it would arise right from the start, when children begin school, and would diminish with each succeeding school year by virtue of the improvement to be expected from conditioning and adaptation.

Frequently a school phobia may appear to arise when a child is emotionally traumatized by an unfeeling teacher or peer. Thus there may be an obvious or visible emotional situation that triggers the onset of the phobic disorder. However, upon deeper examination, one invariably finds evidence of a predisposing dyslexic factor, a factor subconsciously "inviting" teachers and peers to act out unthinking, unfeeling, even sadistic, statements and actions. Occasionally, guilt-ridden dyslexic children and even adults will unconsciously provoke others to abuse or insult them, thereby attempting to satisfy their underlying guilt feelings and a resulting need for punishment. They feel stupid and dumb, disappointments to their parents and teachers—worthless.

Those dyslexics who cannot vent their academic and social frustration and anger turn it upon themselves in the form of self-abuse.

FEARS OF HEIGHTS, BRIDGES, WALKING: IMBALANCE PHOBIAS

What causes fears of heights and bridges, even irrational-seeming thoughts of jumping out of windows, off train platforms, etc.? In retrospect the answer appears simple: imbalance mechanisms resulting from a dysfunctioning inner-ear system!

One does not have to be "klutzy" to avoid phobically "dangerous" situations that provoke inner feelings of imbalance and fear of falling. Dyslexic athletes may experience imbalance and vertigo and fear heights, whereas clumsy dyslexics may not be affected by heights. Although an inner sense of imbalance is crucial to fears of heights and bridges, it is not an absolute determining factor. The specific reaction to this imbalance determines whether one will be fearful, remain fearful, or deny the fear altogether in an attempt to overcompensate by sky diving, mountain climbing, or pursuing some other height-related activity.

Imbalance mechanisms sometimes reveal themselves in anxiety dreams: nightmares about flying, falling, being pushed off a building or bridge or out of a window, etc. In a similar fashion, imbalance mechanisms may trigger these very same fears and thoughts during one's waking hours.

AGORAPHOBIA

Agoraphobia—a fear of leaving home and walking in wide-open spaces—is clearly related to a dysfunctioning inner-ear system. Invariably agoraphobics fear fainting, passing out, losing control, dizziness, and imbalance symptoms. Accordingly an agoraphobic will leave the house and walk across the street only if escorted by a trusted companion, someone to hold on to should something happen.

Analysis of agoraphobics clearly reveals that most feel dizzy when crossing a wide-open space: Open spaces trigger in them feelings of dizziness and imbalance, as well as fears of passing out. They require an escort because of an inner-ear dysfunction, not because they are immature and dependent, as has been commonly thought. Moreover the dizziness quickly triggers anxiety mechanisms, which rapidly escalate. The escalation of anxiety in many phobic patients clearly suggests that the fine-tuning of this danger signal—anxiety—is malfunctioning, and that this malfunction may be inner-ear–related as well.

Agoraphobics feel most comfortable when walking next to a building, a railing, a bench, or a trusted companion—anything or anyone to hold on to, should they suddenly become dizzy, feel off balance and faint, or lose control. Open spaces, especially intersections, offer no visible evidence of support, and accordingly trigger several anxiety-ridden concerns: What would happen to me if I suddenly lost my balance and fell or passed out while cars were zooming by me? Who would take care of me in that situation if I were all alone?

Despite the differing clinical terms, individuals who fear open spaces and individuals who fear heights and bridges share one and the same basic anxiety: a fear of falling. And underlying this anxiety is a common dysfunction: an unstable balancing mechanism.

PERCEPTUAL AND CROWD PHOBIAS

Perhaps you are now curious about the relationship between crowd phobias and dyslexia? I was too!

Dyslexics have reported experiencing sensations of dizziness, imbalance, almost loss of consciousness, while looking at certain wallpaper patterns or designs, book patterns in libraries, can configurations in food stores, clothing patterns in department stores, "moving-people patterns" along New York City's crowded streets. Upon testing a wide range of these dyslexics with my 3-D Optical Scanner, I inadvertently provoked these very same responses. It became apparent that *visual* patterns or crowds may trigger motion sickness and anxiety reactions in a fashion similar to the motion triggers—buses, cars, planes, elevators, escalators, and carnival rides. Moreover these visually triggered symptoms frequently responded very favorably to medications, and the phobia either lessened or disappeared.

Noise patterns, crowds, even smells, may serve to discombobulate some dyslexics. They will avoid parties and restaurants, and hence suffer from social phobias, restaurant phobias, etc.

Water phobias exist as well. Many dyslexics report motion-sickness responses while watching the ocean rolling to the shore. Overly sensitive individuals feel the same way about ripples on a pond. These patterns serve as visual triggers.

Some dyscoordinated dyslexics justifiably fear drowning, for they simply cannot learn the movement patterns necessary for swimming and survival.

SENSORY–DEPRIVATON PHOBIAS

Many dyslexics are afraid of diving or swimming underwater, especially with their eyes closed. One dyslexic patient reported complete disorientation while scuba diving—he could not distinguish up from down. In fact, he almost drowned because he swam downward while thinking he was swimming upward. Only the pressure buildup in his ears made him realize his error and saved his life.

Swimming underwater becomes a problem for some dyslexics only when their eyes are closed. Once under water and in the dark, they become completely confused, disoriented, and frightened; some refuse to swim underwater under any circumstances, while others merely refuse to close their eyes while swimming underwater.

A dyslexic child might become fearful of the dark and even of falling asleep, thus "preferring" insomnia or falling asleep with his eyes open while watching television or reading a book. Dyslexics have reported experiencing severe dizziness upon closing their eyes, especially prior to falling asleep. Others have reported severe dizzy spells only during sleep. As mentioned, some dyslexics report nightmares concerning falling, floating, and spinning.

You are no doubt wondering why and how these symptoms arise. Psychologists were equally curious, which accounts for the wide range of psychological theories to explain these phenomena. However, I frequently found physical mechanisms to be responsible for these symptoms.

As explained in Chapter IX, concentration and eye-fixation *mechanisms* tend to minimize or eliminate dizziness, imbalance, and other inner-ear symptoms. These compensatory inner-ear mechanisms are sharply reduced when swimming underwater with one's eyes closed, when closing one's eyes before falling asleep, and when actually sleeping.

Some individuals are even fearful of being tired, hence they are compulsively driven to get enough sleep; some resort to coffee and drug "regulation." Concentration is significantly reduced with fatigue and may result in significant intensification of dyslexic symptoms as well as fears of losing control, passing out, and disorientation.

Why should dyslexics be frightened of tunnels or experience claustrophobia? This question was the most difficult to answer.

Many dyslexics have reported a dread of being trapped in a room without a window or door for escape. For this reason, many such individuals will not go to a movie unless they can sit close to an exit (movie phobias); they need a way out in case something should happen to them or in the event that they feel threatened by a loss of control. They fear fainting, passing out, losing consciousness, and experiencing escalating degrees of anxiety. They need a visible means of escaping these dreadful feelings should they arise: They need to know that they can escape to the outside.

In other words claustrophobics feel trapped by inescapable inner, "deadly" feelings; they feel better when there is a visible, external way out. When there is no visible way out, it is as if their inner sense of feeling overwhelmed is confirmed externally; their anxiety escalates even further, and they feel even more trapped. Stated another way, their feeling free to escape from their external environment really reflects the need to escape from their inner environment, which often consists of escalating or improperly controlled anxiety or dread. Visible signs of escape are reassuring, whereas the absence of such is devastating.

What do tunnels, moving elevators, closed-off rooms, stationary elevators, and underwater situations have in common, except for the fact that they trigger claustrophobia? As suggested earlier, they are all encircling environments that may be difficult to escape from and thus intensify feelings of being trapped and losing control of one's feelings and anxieties. But why should these environments trigger anxiety in the first place?

One additional thought occurred to me. All of the above situations are *shielding* environments—environments that encircle individuals and completely shut them off from their "normal" surroundings. They appear to be "sensory-deprivation" environments. Is it possible that shielding environments may impair the inner ear's ability to receive and utilize vital electromagnetic and related visual signals needed to maintain and even regain orientation and contact with one's surrounding, especially if the inner ear is already somewhat impaired in these functions?

Dyslexics already have impaired "antennae" secondary to their inner-ear dysfunction. Accordingly, dyslexics receive incoming signals in a partially blurred fashion, but are able to compensate for it. If they pass through a shielding environment, then the signals coming in are further impaired and their "radio" functioning and reception become similar to that of one's car radio when one rides through a tunnel. In a "tunnel," dyslexics' inability to function properly or maintain contact with the outside world may result in severe anxiety and appropriate avoidance mechanisms or phobias.

External Versus Internal Triggers

Before continuing with an explanation of the universal phobias (common phobias that exist, and have always existed, in every society), I must clarify what I mean by external and internal triggers and their corresponding response mechanisms, i.e., phobias.

Thus far the inner-ear–related phobias or phobic mechanisms described were *released* or *triggered* by stimuli. These stimuli are called *external triggers:* cars, buses, planes, trains, elevators, escalators, bridges, heights, and crowds; visual, auditory, and olfactory configurations. Psychoanalysts have viewed these triggers as sexual symbols, indicating that cars, buses, planes, etc., represent aspects of the sexual anatomy and/or intercourse. Perhaps, but not necessarily so.

My research indicates that these triggers may be symbolic only of specific motion stimuli to which an impaired inner-ear system is sensitive and to which it therefore reacts abnormally. In fact, there is significant evidence to suggest that the cerebellum, the computer for the inner-ear system, modulates and regulates anxiety, as well as sexual and aggressive drives and emotions, as it does the other sensory and motor mechanisms. Hence, improper fine-tuning of all these instincts and reflexes may predispose individuals to a corresponding series of sexual and aggressive symptoms. In other words, sexual and aggressive instincts may indeed contribute to the presence of phobias and related mental disorders. However, these instincts, as well as the anxiety mechanisms they trigger, may be impaired primarily by an underlying physiological dysfunction previously overlooked in psychiatric research.

Internal triggers may also provoke abnormal phobic and other responses. Thus, for example, dysfunctioning inner-ear mechanisms may be released by such internal triggers as abnormal chemical states, diabetes, thyroid disease, shifting hormone levels during menses and menopause, tumors, and any other disorder that impairs the function of the cells that are essential to the inner-ear system.

The significance of both external and especially internal triggers in provoking phobias and related mental disorders has been significantly overlooked by both psychiatrists and other medical researchers. The presence of phobias in the absence of any clear-cut physical or neurological disorder has led to the assumption that the released mental symptom is of primary psychological or mental origin, i.e., caused by conflicting emotions. Overlooked was Freud's ingenious insight that underlying all mental and emotional disorders exists a physical component, or "somatic compliance."

Now, to return to the universal phobias . . .

Universal Phobias

Such universal phobias as fears of insects, snakes, knives, etc., have always been known to mankind, regardless of how primitive or complex the society. As might have been expected, these phobias were viewed by psychoanalysts as sexually or aggressively determined, and the corresponding trigger was viewed as having a sexual or aggressive symbolic significance.

The universal phobias I am talking about deliberately exclude realistic or *traumatic phobias*—phobias that result from a real trauma, e.g., being attacked by an animal, bitten by an insect, attacked by a knife or weapon, or sexually and/or aggressively molested and abused. I eventually came to view universal phobias as release symptoms—the release of old, buried fears dating back to our original animal origins and heritage; fears reflecting the instincts and reflexes inherited by animal species for survival over millions and millions of years.

Few of us are fully aware of how inherited reflex patterns are crucial to our survival, and how dependent these reflexes are on triggers. For example, the newborn infant has a sucking reflex once his cheek is touched, a crying reflex when spanked, a breathing reflex that responds to changing oxygen levels in the air and blood, and an eye-tracking reflex provoked by moving visual triggers. All of these reflex motor patterns are inherited. They were imprinted in our genes during an evolutionary process of survival of the fittest.

Animal species are known to have inherited sexual, aggressive, and flight patterns of response to certain external stimuli: colors, scents, noise patterns, and visual configurations, such as the shapes of insects and other animal forms. Humans no longer need many of these inherited response patterns; the response patterns have been neutralized or buried by strong inhibitory mechanisms or counterforces that hold them in check. These antiquated reflex patterns are held controlled or regulated by our central nervous systems unless there is some impairment within the inhibitory forces. In the presence of such an impairment, old, buried fears and anxieties are released from inhibitory control and surface as symptoms of phobias. In other words, currently unnecessary patterns of response may be released from inhibition by triggers that, under normal circumstances, would have no triggering potency. I have frequently observed dyslexics experiencing difficulty with certain motor reflexes—difficulty holding a pen, spooon, or a knife and fork properly—utilizing animallike grasping mechanisms. Some dyslexics have difficulty with reflexes needed to process sound inputs and speech outputs rapidly. Others have difficulty "learning" to blow their noses or swallow pills, i.e., difficulty with coordinated reflex responses. Also, many dyslexics are given to releasing anxiety and motion-sickness responses when triggered by stimuli that do not affect nondyslexic individuals. Thus, many dyslexics display fears of snakes and other animals by which they have never been threatened.

Keeping all of these observations in mind, I reasoned as follows:

- If the inner ear and cerebellum are responsible for coordinating and releasing normal reflexes, and
- If some reflexes are poorly released and poorly coordinated among dyslexics, and
- If some anxiety and motion-sickness release mechanisms are "abnormally" triggered in dyslexics, and

- If the cerebellum or inner-ear system is an "organ" whose prime function is inhibition, according to Nobel prizewinner Sir John Eccles,
- Then might not a dysfunctioning inner-ear or cerebellar system with failure in inhibitory power result in the release of old, primitive instincts, reflexes, i.e., universal phobic responses?

This reasoning can explain how universal phobias may occur without any external trauma or trigger. It also accounts for the universality of these fears and their complete independence of specific patterns of child-rearing and personality profiles.

Incomplete Psychiatric Assumptions

Most clinicians, psychiatric and otherwise, assume that a disorder is psychologically or emotionally determined if physical or physiological factors cannot be found. In the absence of a clearly defined physical basis for a disorder or symptom, psychoanalysts and psychiatrists quite naturally propose the presence of unconscious, unseen, intangible emotional or mental mechanisms. Unfortunately errors have been, and still are being, made.

The absence of detectable physical findings may be due either to faulty clinical examinations or to physicians' inability to detect and recognize the presence of existing physical and physiological dysfunctioning. The entire dyslexic riddle was a consequence of faulty medical assumptions, circular reasoning patterns, incomplete neurological examinations, denial of the presence of inner-ear–related signs and symptoms, and even the imaginary belief in the presence of cortical signs where none existed. The so-called absence of concrete physical factors in dyslexia initially led to the assumption and conviction that this disorder and its various symptoms were psychologically determined. Two factors were found to result in this error:

- The stated absence of tangible, physical signs does not necessarily mean that these signs are really absent, and that they cannot be detected by another clinician, or by newer, more advanced diagnostic medical instruments.
- The assumption and especially the conviction that a symptom or disorder is psychologically determined must be based on more than the absence of physical findings; it must be based on the presence of positive, tangible psychological factors.

Anyone can postulate that psychological mechanisms are responsible for a disorder—even cancer—for which there is no currently established physical cause. However, the mere assumption of a psychological cause does not warrant conviction or psychological treatment until positive supporting evidence is found. My research into phobias and a host of related, so-called emotionally caused disorders led me to recognize that accepted scientific "fact" was, in reality, mere fantasy.

The study of dyslexia and the inner-ear mechanisms responsible for dyslexic symptoms led me to the unexpected but clearly demonstrated physical basis of phobias. Moreover this physical basis was experimentally proven. The fact that phobic symptoms respond favorably to medications administered specifically to improve inner-ear functioning further added to my conviction that the primary cause and basis of phobias is a dysfunctioning inner ear.

Although psychological mechanisms and triggers may provoke phobias that are inner ear related, and although some phobias are entirely due to psychological factors, my research has clearly demonstrated that a majority of the phobias examined to date are clearly not primarily of psychological origin. Psychological mechanisms may, and do, cause non-dyslexic academic symptoms. However, these psychologically determined academic symptoms are different in quality, shape, and form from their dyslexic counterparts, and therefore must be treated differently.

Although there still exists a medical bias against psychological medicine, nonpsychiatric physicians are all too eager to attribute psychological causes and motives to patients' symptoms. Unfortunately psychiatrists and psychologists are similarly inclined to accept these psychological diagnoses without medically double-checking the patients and without clear-cut positive evidence to support a psychological diagnosis.

I have never quite forgotten an episode that occurred during my psychiatric residency at Kings County Hospital in Brooklyn, New York. While working in the psychiatric admitting room, a confused, disoriented young man was transferred to me from the medical emergency room. Although inexperienced psychiatrically during my first year of residency, I sensed the man's confusion was not of psychological origin. Despite his having been cleared medically, I reexamined him neurologically and found him to have suspiciously abnormal signs suggesting a brain dysfunction.

As a result of my examination, I called the medical emergency room, told the referring medical residents what I thought, and refused to accept the patient for admission to a psychiatric ward despite his loud verbal ramblings, and disturbing behavior. A conflict inevitably resulted between the residents in the emergency room and me. The patient was transferred back to the medical emergency room. My superior was contacted and a telephone argument resulted and lasted for hours, with time out on both sides to examine new patients. By morning the patient settled the argument: He developed a temperature of 104 degrees, became increasingly incoherent, and developed clear-cut, irrefutable signs of an infection of his nervous system. Despite antibiotics and rigorous treatment efforts, he died of a rare infectious disease of the nervous system.

Although my diagnostic abilities are far from perfect, and I have had my share of unfortunate errors, my reasoning remains sound: Assumptions are only assumptions, regardless of the individuals making them, and traditionally accepted convictions without logic and without proof are still only assumptions.

Earlier in my career, some of the psychoanalytical literature on phobias and related mental functioning just never sat well with me despite my repeated attempts to read and reread the content for better understanding and conviction. However, when in doubt, especially when inexperienced, it is often best to suspend judgment until increasing clinical experience allows for realistic and more sound reappraisals.

Following my realization that a majority of phobias are physically based and shaped by inner-ear mechanisms, I once again reread *The Psychoanalytic Theory of Neurosis* by one of the most outstanding analysts in the history of the psychoanalytic movement, Otto Fenichel. Lo and behold, there was a written correlation between phobias, hysteria, dizziness, and a tendency toward motion sickness. There was just one rub: Fenichel believed the inner-ear symptoms were a result of the phobias and anxiety.* I had demonstrated the opposite to be true. The inner-ear symptoms of dizziness, equilibrium sensations, and motion sickness correlate with phobias solely because all four symptoms are directly related to and caused by an inner-ear dysfunction.

According to classic psychoanalytical theory, if a student or patient can't *see, feel,* and meaningfully *accept* stated analytical facts, then these students or patients must be defensively resisting this acceptance because of unconscious emotional factors and conflicts. But this is not necessarily so.

To test my own inner-ear theory of phobias, I examined all my phobic patients with my 3-D Optical Scanner for inner-ear dysfunction. All phobics tested were found to have abnormally low blurring speeds, in-

*See Fenichel's argument in Appendix C.

dicative of a dysfunctioning inner ear. Moreover, all such patients were questioned about past evidence of dyslexic symptoms. All patients revealed clear signs and symptoms of dyslexia.

In addition, a significant number of treated dyslexics revealed improvement in phobic symptoms, a finding highly consistent with my inner-ear theory and inconsistent with traditional analytical theory. I then began treating phobic patients with the same medications I successfully used to treat dyslexia. Many of these phobics suddenly and dramatically showed signs of improvement—improvement that did not occur when treated by me psychiatrically.

In summary, over a period of many years I recognized the relationship between phobias and the inner-ear from two seemingly independent lines of research:

(1) The vast majority of phobias psychiatrically examined and psychotherapeutically treated could neither be successfully explained nor helped by utilizing traditional analytical theories. Something crucial was missing.
(2) Dyslexic children and adults were frequently noted to display a series of motion-related, compass-related, academic-related, and balance-and-coordination–related phobias identical to those seen in a typical psychiatric practice. These dyslexia-related phobias could be physiologically and psychologically explained and better treated utilizing anti–motion-sickness medications.

To highlight the correlation between dyslexia, inner-ear dysfunction, and phobias, a series of phobic cases will be presented. Analyze their content and judge for yourself.

11
Phobias—Case Histories

IN WRITING THIS CHAPTER, I HAVE TRIED TO PRESENT THE clinical content in a manner and sequence similar to the way I experienced it. However, for the sake of clarity, I was forced to group and organize the clinical data so that its meaning and significance would be more readily apparent.

Although puzzles and riddles are fascinating to solve, who would have published this book if the data were presented as they first appeared to me: random and seemingly disconnected, scrambled, and "dyslexic"? In the preceding chapter, "Phobias and the Inner Ear," I presented the theories that I found useful in explaining and better organizing a confusing array of phobic symptoms that appeared completely independent of and separated from one another, except by name. In retrospect, these seemingly disconnected clinical phobic syndromes no longer appear scrambled, blurry, and confusing. In fact, the vast variety of phobic symptoms have now been readily united under a common theoretical cause: the inner ear.

Phobias have always cropped up in dyslexic case histories. However, no one seemed to pay these symptoms any attention. In other words they were blocked out of scientific view by bias, i.e., scientifically denied.

The reverse was true as well. Dyslexic symptoms have invariably characterized phobic cases in psychiatric treatment. Unfortunately these dyslexic symptoms were completely overlooked. Once again scientific bias was found to be responsible for this amazing oversight.

As a result of my research, the presence of phobias in dyslexia, and the frequency of dyslexia among phobics, can no longer be denied or scientifically "blurred out." Phobias are part and parcel of the dyslexic disorder and are caused by the same dysfunction.

One aim of this chapter is to introduce you to some of my phobic patients. After reading, hearing, and feeling their thoughts and experiences, try to dissect the separate but interwoven psychological and physiological factors that determine and shape their various symptoms. Form your own theories.

Initially, I had no idea that my psychiatric phobic patients were dyslexic despite their being under my psychotherapeutic care for many years. I was merely interested in psychologically treating their symptoms by listening to their free associations and then explaining and resolving their *assumed* emotional conflicts. My phobic patients *never* hinted at dyslexic symptoms until specifically questioned for them despite years of careful psychiatric observations. This experience clearly suggested to me that all psychiatric patients must be actively questioned and examined for symptoms. Waiting for psychiatric patients to verbalize their problems spontaneously and freely may result in wasted years and misdiagnoses.

Slowly and unexpectedly I came to realize that the phobias displayed by psychiatric patients were similar, then identical, to those revealed to me by dyslexic children and adults. Slowly, I came to recognize that dyslexic phobias improved and even disappeared when dyslexic patients were treated with anti–motion-sickness medications. (Remember: No one should treat himself, even with over-the-counter medications.)

This chapter will carry these insights a giant step forward and show you a validated new method of understanding, diagnosing, and treating phobias of inner-ear origin. Furthermore the cases to be presented will allow you to test my theories as well as any you may have formulated on your own.

Recently Diagnosed and Treated Phobics—Case Histories

MARGARITA MAGARO

Margarita, an attractive thirty-seven-year-old flight attendant, was examined by me for phobias and other symptoms that had been plaguing her for some time. These phobias were:

- Fear of crossing streets
- Fear of being alone in a strange city
- Fear of skiing, a sport she had once loved and in which she had excelled
- Fear of making decisions.

Margarita also suffered from:

- Dizziness, particularly when turning to the right
- Fatigue
- Blurred and fuzzy vision most of the time
- Poor handwriting ability
- Memory instability for names, dates, and numbers
- Reading and concentration difficulties since childhood
- Chronic confusion with regard to where she was.

In spite of these difficulties or because of them, she chose to be a flight attendant.

When I asked Margarita to tell me about her symptoms, she replied:

I am dreadfully afraid to make mistakes when I am asked to read something, particularly in the presence of others. I cross my eyes and say I am unable to see, deliberately making myself "blind" to justify my statement.

I cannot make a decision. I think first one way and then another, and finally I make up my mind at the last possible moment.

. . . It is the same when I have chores to do. I wait until I can no longer procrastinate. It's terrible.

And . . . permeating these actions, there is an all-pervasive sense of anxiety and fear that has become worse and worse.

Examination revealed that Margarita's phobias and related symptoms were due to a dysfunctioning inner-ear system. Accordingly she was placed on medication. Shortly afterward she wrote to me excitedly:

Everything looks and feels so crisp and fresh! I am calmer, more in control of myself, able to make judgments and arrive at decisions. *No more procrastinating!*

I'm feeling no more anxiety or fear—it is all easier. I can drive a car with assurance, play tennis, and I have vacationed alone for the first time in twelve years!

Also, I'm unbelievably better organized! One week after being on medication, I returned home and was shocked to see the disorganized, messy state of my house. I went through the house and garage, cleaning, discarding, and reorganizing like mad. Just as my chaotic, messy house reflected the old me, it now reflects the new me. It is uncluttered, purposeful, fresh, and bright.

Margarita is euphoric about her newfound freedom. Although she wrote the following words, I can imagine her saying them with her intriguing, charming Italian accent: "I hope that my ability to cope will give me more energy and time to devote to others. . . . Thank you."

ANNE MASSIE

Very often parents seek help for their children and inadvertently find help for themselves. This was the case with Anne Massie.

Anne had brought her son Tom for treatment and he had responded extremely well. Anne then sought help for herself: She was suffering from incapacitating phobias that were destroying her way of life, as well as deeply upsetting her loved ones. Anne's phobias were:

- Fear of talking to people because the words might come out backward or might not come out at all
- Fear of speaking on the telephone
- Fear of driving on the freeway
- Fear of the water
- Fear of heights.

Initially, Anne denied or "forgot" having had academic problems in grammar school. She was not able to read and she recalled fooling her mother and teachers by memorizing the words on the page. She could not properly recognize the words she tried to read. As she became older she learned to read despite the persistence of letter and word reversals and a resulting memory instability for what she read. Right/left directional difficulties persisted into adulthood.

Although not a very good student, Anne managed to pass her courses. She related the following paradoxical pattern of good versus poor coordination skills:

On two separate occasions I climbed a tree and then had to be rescued because I was afraid of falling. I never went climbing again.

Although I was a poor dancer, I was an excellent horseback rider. I loved horses and riding.

I was very artistic and earned my living as a painter. Yet, my writing was never really neat.

Anne continued:

I married and had two beautiful children. The marriage, however, did not work out and we got divorced. I supported my children and myself with my portrait painting.

My ex-husband then took our children to South America.

I almost went out of my mind, I was devastated.

I was unable to get my children back. I was unable to paint. . . . I went into analysis, which did help. Then I met a wonderful man whose love and understanding attracted me. We married and had a son, who has filled our lives with joy. Both of my other children were never far from my thoughts. I can only hope that when they are ready, they will seek me out.

Anne's extreme disappointment over losing her children, over not being able to establish personal contact with them, and over the realization that she could do nothing more until they were ready to see her triggered a series of phobias that increased in severity and number over a period of years.

I had become afraid to talk to people. I feared the words would come out backward or not come out at all. And I feared sounding and appearing stupid. I reached the point where I avoided speaking on the telephone. My mind would blank out . . . I could not get the words out. Eventually the ringing of the telephone was enough for panic to set in. It was terrible.

I had always driven on the freeway without any difficulty. Suddenly I was frightened to do so. My fears extended to include heights. I was an excellent swimmer and enjoyed the water. But [then] I became mortally afraid of the water.

I developed headaches that became more and more frequent and intense, increasing my sense of confusion, anxiety, and inadequacy. I had become so depressed and isolated that I was almost unable to function.

It was our son, Tom, whose need gave me the strength to come to Dr. Levinson's office and ultimately to receive help for us both.

Anne was examined, diagnosed as dyslexic with associated phobias, and placed on medication.

Tom's and Anne's progress reports indicated a turnaround for both. On a visit a year later, Dr. Massie, Anne's husband, commented on their son's improvement:

Undeniable and unreal! We note progress in his speech, concentration, memory, reading, and writing—better spacing between letters, and coordination. Before our visit Tom would have never entertained the thought of tennis lessons. Recently he not only took tennis lessons, but they have revealed an aptitude for the game! He is playing with experienced players and handling himself very creditably. You can't imagine what this has done for his confidence.

Tom now has many newfound relationships with others of his own age. We are so pleased at his progress.

In no way can we attribute this improvement to coincidence or any other factor but your correct diagnosis and treatment. We are grateful.

I thanked Dr. Massie and then questioned Anne about the changes she had noticed in herself this past year.

I am painting again after fifteen years! And I have sold several paintings already. This is a marvelously heady feeling for me!

I have friends that I enjoy talking to, both in person and *on the telephone*! No longer does the ring of the phone and the possibility of answering the phone strike terror in me.

I drive on the freeway once again; it is no longer a fearful vortex, sucking me into its center and oblivion. . . .

This summer I have gone *swimming*—can you believe it? Once again I am able to enjoy the sport and the water.

My whole world has changed. The shadows are gone and the colors are bold and bright. I have more energy, fewer headaches. I can concentrate and organize my thoughts and activities without going into a tailspin. I feel more self-confident and better about myself as a person.

My memory still leaves something to be desired; I forget names and regress somewhat under stress, but these are slight drawbacks.

I feel an improvement in almost every area, especially inside. There is an inner calm and stability; I feel almost reborn.

Anne's improved self-concept and general feeling of well-being spring from her achievements and joy, not only in her progress, but in her son's as well. Her case clearly indicates how emotional stress and conflict may trigger a disruption within a preexisting compensated but impaired inner-ear system, and thus the emergence or reemergence of dyslexic and phobic symptoms.

It must be emphasized that although emotional stress and conflict were triggers, they did not cause, create, or shape the *forms* of the resulting phobic symptoms. The forms of the phobic symptoms were determined by the pattern of impaired inner-ear mechanisms. Accordingly the resulting phobic symptoms improved when the underlying mechanisms responded favorably to medications improving inner-ear functions and mechanisms. What's more, the fact that Anne was a poor dancer and a superb rider highlights two major physiological factors:

- Each and every motor and sensory function is controlled or processed by its own corresponding channel; thus athletes may be gifted for one motor task and klutzy for another.
- Interest and concentration are potent compensatory factors that are often crucial in leading to improved inner-ear functioning.

SUSAN SMITH

Seeing Susan's perpetual smile, one would never guess that she was the victim of severe, paralyzing phobias and assorted dyslexic symptoms.

For many years Susan suffered from:

- Fear of crossing streets
- Fear of becoming lost
- Fear of riding escalators
- Fear of going on elevators alone
- Fear of driving and of being in cars
- Fear of being in the city alone
- Fear of heights, which resulted in avoidance of bridges, cable cars, tunnels, etc.
- Fear of water and of drowning.

Other symptoms were:

- Poor sense of time
- Poor sense of direction, and right/left difficulty
- Clumsiness.

Susan's many problems clearly illustrated the interwoven nature of phobias and related dyslexic symptoms. The following is an excerpt from our discussion:

"As a child, I had a lot of trouble staying upright. I was falling constantly. I tried roller skating and ended up on my backside most of the time. I was falling, tripping, and bumping into things and people; it was terribly humiliating.

"I was extremely afraid of crossing streets. My mother was still picking me up at school, helping me cross the street, etc., even when I was quite old. When I crossed on my own, I was afraid of being struck by a car because I had no idea where the cars were coming from. I was confused: I didn't know whether to cross the street when the light was red, as my mother told me to do, or to cross when the light was green, as my teacher advised. What I ended up doing was running across the street and praying a lot.

"In retrospect I think my mother was confused too. I recall that she had trouble crossing the streets. We'd start crossing, a car would come, she would go back, the car would start, she would go forward, the car would stop—it was like a dance. Whenever a car approached, she would just stop. I did the same thing, I guess, and a couple of times I was almost killed.

"When I walked, I always crossed the street at the narrowest place. If it was a quiet street or a narrow one, it was okay, but if it was a busy or very wide street, I had a problem. I would simply wait until there were no cars. After I had my baby daughter, I virtually stopped crossing streets. I felt responsible for her, so I didn't go anywhere. I walked around the block or went to the park, where I could sit.

"I was always very apprehensive about escalators and elevators. With my husband or friends I would go up the escalator but never down. I was terrified of falling. Actually, I feared that my foot might become caught on the step; I would panic, become light-headed. For years my therapist worked with me through behavior therapy and desensitization. I was finally able to go down escalators, but with great difficulty and fear. It created a problem when my husband and I went out: We always had to find an elevator.

"I was afraid of riding in an elevator unless someone was with me; I was afraid the door would crush me. Actually it's always been like that: If I'm with somebody, my husband or a friend, I give them the responsibility of taking care of me and protecting me.

"My therapist showed me how to hold the door of the elevator open so that it wouldn't close. I became better as long as I could hold the door open. I felt it couldn't crush me and I would be okay. If for some reason I can't control the door and keep it open until I step in safely, I start to panic and scream; I can't help it. I am also afraid of riding the subway or a train for the same reason: I am afraid of the door closing on me and crushing me.

"I was always afraid of becoming lost. When I began college, I generally got lost. Inadvertently, I would take the wrong buses and would have to ask people for directions; it was a nightmare. That's one of the reasons I dropped out of school. I was phobic, particularly about Manhattan: I was and still am afraid of getting lost there.

"Early in our marriage my husband tried to teach me how to drive and I just couldn't learn. Whenever I was in a car, I believed the other cars would crash headlong into us. I wasn't able to judge how far away the cars were; it's slightly better now, but I do close my eyes and fall asleep. Perhaps it's a way of escaping.

"I was also terrified of bridges and looking down. I was afraid of cable cars too. I wouldn't look down; I didn't want to know that I was that high up and that I might fall off.

"As a child, it was difficult for me in other ways too. I was terrified of my father. He was a very bright man, although not educated. He valued education and brightness. My sister was very, very bright: Her IQ was around genius level, and she didn't have the problems that I had. My father kept telling me that she was smart but that I was kind of dopey. So his whole life was really invested in my sister's being bright, and he kind of gave up on me.

"From the beginning I was a disappointment to him; he had wanted a boy—he made that very clear. He would send me to get things for him, but I never seemed to get what he wanted. Particularly, I dreaded his sending me to his car to get his business books. He would go into great detail describing which books he wanted and their location in the trunk of his car, but I had no idea what he was saying. I couldn't open the trunk, or I would mix the keys up. I would stand there in the street, sweating, because I was so afraid of him. He had a violent temper. If by chance I got the trunk opened, I couldn't tell which side was right and which was left. It was horrible.

"My father insisted I take piano lessons, and he would make me practice in front of him every night. I faked it. I read the music for the right hand pretty well, but not the music for the left hand. It was a disaster. The last piano teacher I had told him he was wasting his money. I knew I was a big disappointment to him.

"I've always had a problem with time. I'm always late because I'm very slow, partly because I drop things constantly. I never seem to allow enough time; my judgment is off. If I have company, I invite them at a certain time, but I'm never ready. I don't mean to be late. I just have no conception of time: I don't know if it's months or years since a particular event; I can't remember. I just have very little time sense.

"The same thing with being clumsy. I've always been klutzy and people have always laughed at me. I learned to make fun of myself. That way I developed a good sense of humor and had lots of friends.

"Due to all my fears, I became very overprotective of my daughter. I wouldn't allow her to ride a bicycle or roller skate because I was afraid she would hurt herself. It was hard for both of us. As a result, I saw a psychiatric social worker about this problem. Later, I began to see the psychiatrist in behavior modification therapy. After years of my being in therapy, he began to think I might have a learning disability. He had been teaching me to cross the streets, and he came to realize that I had no idea from which direction cars were coming—they could have come from the sky as far as I was concerned.

"Then I heard you speak on TV, Dr. Levinson. I thought, Oh, my god, he really knows. I read your book and knew I had to see you."

Susan left my offices with a definite diagnosis of dyslexia and a program of treatment to follow. After years of thinking of herself as klutzy and not too smart and having to battle her different phobias daily, Susan now feels tremendous relief, knowing that she has a physical problem with a prescribed treatment. She is not crazy or stupid.

RITA DROWN

Rita, age twenty-six, suddenly experienced weird sensations while visiting a museum and looking at the paintings on exhibit. The ground beneath her suddenly seemed to shift, and the strange feeling intensified while walking, making her feel uneasy and unsteady—off balance. Moving her head downward or sideways triggered feelings of disorientation and intensified her imbalance and dizziness. Complete concentration was needed to prevent swaying, falling, or tripping. Needless to say, she became frightened and upset about these symptoms.

Rita visited one of the most prominent neurologists. His examination revealed "absent signs of disease of the nervous system—no signs of vestibular or proprioceptive dysfunction." Although Rita denied feelings of anxiety and tension or personal marital or emotional conflict, the doctor nevertheless diagnosed her as suffering from "neurotic trends."

New symptoms continued to develop. In her mind, objects appeared to turn or spin, whereas external situations remained stationary or merely tilted or angled. Feelings of nausea occurred and began to intensify. Dizziness and light-headedness resulted while walking significant distances. The ground beneath her felt "soft" and "mushy," as though she were walking on a mattress. She suddenly began to fear walking across wide-open spaces (agoraphobia).

As a result of increased symptoms, Rita consulted a noted and well-respected ear, nose, and throat specialist. After a complete physical examination, including an ENG, the specialist concluded that Rita's symptoms were probably of an emotional nature, due to anxiety and tension states.

Rita's symptoms tended to oscillate with time, remitting and intensifying unexplainably. New symptoms developed. Her vision periodically became blurry. She began to fear choking when she ate. Her agoraphobia intensified. She consulted another gifted neurologist. In his report, he stated she was suffering from a subtle disturbance of the integration of eye movements, body balancing and the stabilization of the visual fields.

He said this was presumably due to a disturbance of the brain stem–visual cortex circuits. He found there was no history of a disease process . . . no multiple sclerosis. He further reported that Rita had gone through a period of great difficulty with reading. However, he noted a recent alteration in her glasses seemed to improve that problem. Although this doctor correctly determined the site and physiology of Rita's disturbance, the relationship of these symptoms to her preexisting but hidden dyslexic disorder was not recognized.

Rita's symptoms persisted. She could not accept or understand the contradictory explanations given her. There was no meaningful help. Psychiatric treatment was frequently recommended. She continued to seek help from an endless series of psychiatric and nonpsychiatric physicians.

Following examination, a prominent group of specialists at a famous clinic concluded that Rita's disorder was emotionally based. She was advised to vacation and rest. Upon returning from a rest vacation in Florida, her symptoms suddenly returned in full force. She stopped eating because she was afraid that she would choke while swallowing her food. She lost fifteen pounds. She became increasingly fearful of venturing from home unless accompanied by a trusted companion.

Having read of my research with academic and phobic disturbances, Rita sought my help. Questioning revealed a series of additional symptoms: She had difficulty concentrating and remembering the sequence of the words she wished to say, as if her brain were slowing down. Objects were seen as tilted, and people moving were noted to bob up and down and vibrate from side to side unless she restricted her eye movements. She could not maintain eye contact while talking to someone without becoming severely dizzy. If she looked to the side, it was easier for her to understand what was said, and at the same time she prevented blurred and oscillating vision.

In addition, she spontaneously revealed having had severe math and directional difficulties when younger.

Neurological and physiological eye tracking and ENG testing clearly revealed evidence of an obvious severe inner-ear dysfunction, supporting the second neurologist's findings.

Unfortunately, Rita's confusing and frustrating experience with clinicians and their resulting diagnostic conflicts is typical. Physicians frequently overlook or deny obvious inner-ear signs and symptoms and are all too ready to diagnose misunderstood but typical inner-ear symptoms as "neurotic."

Beware! Pay heed to three basic facts of medical-psychiatric life:

• The absence of medical findings by no means warrants the conclusion and conviction that these undetected findings are not there!

• The absence of medical findings does not justify the conviction that the patient's symptoms are neurotic.

• The diagnosis of neurosis by physicians is merely an *assumption* unless one can clearly demonstrate and prove a psychologically determined cause-and-effect relationship between hidden, unconscious conflicts and resulting symptoms. Moreover the assumed neurotic cause must be able to explain completely the shape and form of the symptoms as well as their onset, remission, and variations.

No doubt some readers are wondering: Did Rita favorably respond to medical treatment? The answer is no: She did not benefit from two trials of prescribed antihistamines and gave up. However, the understanding provided by my diagnosis and explanations facilitated her gaining a measure of control that she did not have before. She could compensate better and avoid provoking physiological and even psychological triggers.

Rita might have benefited from an exploratory trial of psychotherapy. This trial would have aimed at uncovering possible hidden conflicts and relieving them, thus minimizing or eliminating the emotional triggering of her inner-ear dysfunction. However, she was not interested in this exploratory procedure.

Summary

A wide-ranging series of phobias has been presented so that the reader may experience and "see" the clinical content needed to comprehend fully the complex but fascinating relationship between phobias and the inner-ear.

There have been chapters and books written on phobias. Most often the reader is *told,* rather than shown, the cause-and-effect relationships determining phobic symptoms. My phobic theories are derived entirely from the insights provided by my many patients. I thought it only fair to share these patients and their insights with you.

Although all inner-ear–related phobias share an underlying common denominator, each case has its own characteristics and thus requires a correspondingly unique understanding if appropriate diagnosis and treatment are to be effective. In many ways the clinical variations seen among phobics mirror those seen among dyslexics.

These variations were found to be caused by a complex equilibrium consisting of dysfunctioning versus compensatory forces utilizing very specific combinations of physiological circuits. Thus children with poor reading ability may become compulsive readers, and children and adults fearful of heights may eventually become sky divers. Just as dyslexic symptoms may be intensified or reinforced by the development of emotional scarring, the same is true for inner-ear–determined phobic symptoms. Thus any attempt to treat these "mixed" physiological-emotional disorders only with medicines, or only with psychoanalysis, or only with conditioning, is simplistic.

One needs a *holistic* diagnostic-therapeutic approach to phobias that is identical to that needed for dyslexics. I truly hope that the theoretical and clinical insights provided in chapters X and XI will catalyze a new beginning in understanding and treating phobias and related "emotional" disorders physiologically *and* psychologically—holistically.

Predictably the new insights derived from my study of phobias and the inner ear have added incredibly exciting dimensions to my earlier concepts of both dyslexia and phobias:

- The symptomatic horizons of dyslexia have been dramatically expanded, encompassing a wide range of phobias and related emotional symptoms never before conceived of as part of the dyslexic syndrome.
- The physiological basis for phobias and related mental disorders—"somatic compliance"—suddenly materialized into scientific consciousness.
- For the very first time, the physical basis of "mental disorders" could be seen, explored, diagnosed, and understood.
- For the very first time, devastating phobic disorders could be holistically conceptualized and treated utilizing a combined medical-psychological approach.
- For the very first time, patients could be told the real physical meaning and significance underlying and determining their phobic and related mental symptoms, thereby minimizing their self-accusations and feelings of hopelessness, stupidity, and ugliness.
- For the very first time, psychiatry, psychology, and psychoanalysis were united with their physically determined neurological origins.

Perhaps you would like to pause here for a moment and reflect. There is certainly a wealth of exciting new content to be properly assimilated and digested. The insights and clinical content thus far presented represent a new scientific beginning. Feel your way around.

I hope that the remaining chapters will spark your curiosity and excite you, for I will present a series of dyslexic success stories, each highlighting new and undreamed-of accomplishments by people with the disorder dyslexia.

12
Successful Despite Dyslexia

THE NAMES OF SUCH FAMOUS DYSLEXICS AS EDISON, EINstein, Nelson A. Rockefeller, and Patton have been frequently mentioned in books and magazine articles and on television and radio. However, little is really known about their inner feelings and dyslexic symptoms.

In this chapter I will portray the lives of successful dyslexics and those of their dyslexic family members, as well as describe their responses to treatment. I have examined dyslexic physicians, scientists, writers, artists, teachers, engineers, and architects. All had become successful despite their dyslexic disorder.

With proper determination, intelligence, and guidance, many dyslexics have succeeded long before I ever treated them. In fact, many dyslexics would never have succeeded were it not for their need to prove to others—and themselves—that they were not stupid, worthless, and incompetent. In other words, their dyslexia served as a motivation to succeed.

It is anticipated that the following case histories and favorable responses to treatment will bring new hope to and trigger a realistic optimism in all dyslexics and all parents, teachers, and clinicians trying to guide dyslexics to success, even fame.

DR. WALKER

Age: Eighty years
Problems: Stuttering, balance/coordination

MRS. LINDA THOMPSON

Age: Thirty-one years
Problems: Word insertions, focusing difficulties, apprehensions/phobias

STACY THOMPSON

Age: Thirteen years
Problems: School-related

It is not too often that one has the opportunity to examine and treat three generations of the same family. However, this did occur when Mrs. Thompson and her daughter Stacy visited my offices. Shortly afterward Dr. Walker, Mrs. Thompson's father, also came to my Medical Dyslexic Treatment Center.

Mrs. Thompson is a successful businesswoman. Her father was and still is, at eighty years of age, a successful dentist.

When I questioned Mrs. Thompson about her symptoms, she responded that from the time she was a child, she had always felt different from others, but she never understood the nature of her differences. However, when Stacy exhibited similar difficulties, Mrs. Thompson was very concerned and anxious to help her: "I was viewing TV and saw you, Dr. Levinson. To my amazement you were describing the precise symptoms that I had lived with all my life—symptoms and feelings that I had never confided to a living soul. These symptoms were:

• *Word insertions*—adding words that have nothing to do with what I was stating or writing. The questioning glances of others when these incidents occurred made me embarrassed. What was worse, I didn't know why I said what I did. Therefore, when I was around others or in a group of strangers, I was very quiet. If I were to speak to someone face to face, I felt extremely uncomfortable and unconsciously held myself rigidly.

• *Apprehension*—associated with heights, bridges, and escalators. Despite a love of skiing, I have felt anxious and apprehensive whenever I looked down a slope or mountain.

- *Angulation and drifting of words/letters off a page* when writing, even though the page was lined.

- *Difficulty in writing down an idea or a thought.* By the time I would get started, the idea would be gone. It was infuriating!

- *Focusing problem.* When driving, particularly at night or when I was tired, I found that I would turn my head to one side in order to see properly.

"I seemed to have all the symptoms you described. . . . I quickly called my husband into the room to listen to your discussion. I was shocked to learn that these symptoms were part of the disorder known as dyslexia. I had never even heard of it before, let alone known I had it. I realized that my daughter Stacy, so like me, probably had the same disorder.

"Stacy was experiencing failures and problems in school. Although a bright, outgoing child, she thought of herself as stupid because she had academic difficulties associated with reading, writing, math, etc. Not even her friendliness, athletic agility, and eager-to-please mannerisms softened the blow of being different from her friends. Her need to study longer in order to learn, only to forget quickly what she had learned, her poor performance on tests—all reinforced her feelings of inadequacy and stupidity.

"Stacy and I sometimes spoke for hours about her problems and feelings. To help ease her pain, I revealed the difficulties that I had experienced in school and when I took tests. I told her that I had wanted so badly to be liked by my peers that I would often do favors, even the laundry, for my friends when I attended college.

"However, once I put aside my books and no longer needed to take tests, everything became easier. My innate abilities and strong desire to succeed took over, and I forged ahead. 'Your father and I have built a successful oceanography business. I succeeded because of, or in spite of, my difficulties. This will happen to you, too, Stacy,' I said.

"I wanted so much to infuse her with self-confidence and an appreciation of the things she could do. What I told her helped—only temporarily, however. With your appearance and discussion on the show, I thought, Perhaps now I can do something of more permanent value for Stacy.

"My husband and I picked her up at camp, and excitedly I told her about our scheduled appointments at your Medical Dyslexic Treatment Center. She listened attentively and hopefully."

Stacy and her mother were examined. Both were found to be dyslexic. An individualized regime of medication was prescribed for each. The

Thompsons felt improvement. They urged Dr. Walker, Mrs. Thompson's father, to seek consultation, too, for the problem of stuttering, which he had had most of his life, and for a difficulty with coordination that he had recently acquired. He came and was also diagnosed as dyslexic. Treatment was prescribed.

Two years later the Thompsons came from Canada for a revisit. The thirteen-year-old young lady who sat across from me was happy and excited to tell me about all the wonderful new changes in her life.

"Before I saw you, Dr. Levinson, and was put on medication, I was either failing my courses or just about passing them," Stacy said. "Now I am getting A's and B's—it's incredible! I just can't believe it! I used to feel different, dumb, afraid no one would like me.

"I wanted so much to be liked by the girls that I would buy them things or do favors for them. I was never sure if it was me they really liked or the things I did for them. Now I'm myself, and if someone doesn't like me, I can deal with it. It's no longer as important as it once was.

"I always loved to draw. But I draw better now than ever before. I also find that I ski, race, and play tennis much, much better than I ever did. My coordination and balance are better and I feel wonderful!"

Extremely pleased with Stacy's progress, I turned my attention to Mrs. Thompson. She, too, looked happier and less tense and anxious than during our last visit.

"My difficulties with expressing myself—those word insertions—are a thing of the past," Mrs. Thompson stated. "Also, I feel more comfortable conversing with others; I'm still not the chattiest person at a gathering, but I'm no longer the most quiet either. I even communicate more with my husband. I've said more to him these past two years than I did in all the years we have been married up until then. He's amazed at the change.

"I always used a Dictaphone in business because I wanted to be sure all my ideas and thoughts were recorded. I also preferred using the telephone so that I would not have to speak face-to-face with a customer. However, I am now able to converse face-to-face without discomfort. Also, I can synchronize my thoughts and my writing: No longer must I use the Dictaphone to be sure I don't lose an idea.

"Driving is also much easier. I can focus better and no longer do I turn my head sideways to see better.

"Skiing, a sport the entire family enjoys, is a lot more fun these days too. I do not feel apprehensive when I am at the top of a slope or mountain. I just take off without a twinge of anxiety!

"Last year, my husband and I went to Scotland. Although we had been there before, I marveled at the countryside. The flowers and foliage were gorgeous; the purples, whites, and blues were breathtaking. I did not remember them as having the sharpness, vividness, and clarity that I saw now. Even my husband was surprised by my reactions. I felt as though scales had been removed from my eyes.

"The anxiety that I previously experienced whenever I was on a bridge or escalator or in any situation where heights are involved is no longer present. All in all, we have come a long way, Stacy and I.

"My father, too, has experienced good results. Can you believe it? At age eighty-two he no longer stutters—after a lifetime of stuttering!

"His balance is also much improved. He no longer trips or stumbles at the least provocation. Every day he walks one to two miles—without his cane.

"Recently he had a cataract operation. As a result of the operation and the medication, his vision is 20/20. He says that he can see more clearly and better than he ever did in his whole life. He says, 'Too bad that I have this old chassis. I feel so good inside!'

"This past year I visited my parents at their home in Indiana. It was the first time that I had seen my father since he started taking medication for his dyslexic symptoms. We spent a wonderful afternoon together, conversing in a manner that we had never before enjoyed. Previously, if we talked, it was only for a few moments: He would be off to do one thing or another. I learned little things about my dad that afternoon that I never knew. He never used to sit long enough for us to share much of ourselves. What a shame, but I shall always be grateful for those precious moments we spent together that day."

Both Dr. Walker and Mrs. Thompson are examples of people who have achieved success despite having dyslexia.

Dr. Walker ran away from home at the tender age of thirteen at the time of his mother's death. He worked at odd jobs to support himself. When he was twenty years old he married a registered nurse. No doubt her influence and his desire to make something of himself motivated him to return to school. He worked and attended high school, college, and then dental school. Despite the Depression, a family to support, and his dyslexia, he succeeded in becoming a successful dentist. His wife was always very supportive and helped him in every way.

Dr. Walker is a very successful man, truly young in heart and spirit. He does orthodontic work for those children whose parents are unable to afford the services of an orthodontist. He derives tremendous gratification from helping these youngsters.

SUSAN STAFFORD

Age: Twenty-four years
Problems: Reading, spelling, coordination, and concentration

"The large number of children who experience school phobias and the number of academic difficulties many children experience motivated me to enter the field of special education. Everything I read in the field convinced me the experts were missing something crucial. Accepted theories about learning disabilities and dyslexia did not sufficiently explain the scope and complexity of the disorder.

"I could not subscribe to the view that the cerebral cortex was the site of the problem. These theories did not make any sense to me. . . .

"The reason I felt so strongly about this is that I am dyslexic. Although I have reading and spelling problems, I score high on differential aptitude tests for abstract and mechanical reasoning. Obviously someone with brain damage could not have a high score in abstract reasoning and math.

"Since I felt the data on learning disabilities was insufficient and certainly not helping dyslexic children to deal with school-related and other problems, I decided to enter the field of research in special education and put my firsthand experience and learning to good use."

These are the sentiments of vivacious, bright Sue Stafford, a graduate student in special education. My first impulse was to congratulate her for her honest, open, and straightforward thinking. Young learning-disability teachers with firsthand dyslexic experience, armed with the latest scientific knowledge, could significantly make a difference where it counts—in the classroom. The driving force behind my years of research has been to help dyslexic children medically and to promote understanding and proper guidance among teachers, parents, and clinicians. Between medical treatment and an emotionally supportive environment in the classroom, children can be spared the humiliating and debilitating effects of dyslexia.

Concerned and knowledgeable teachers and educators are vitally needed. Medication is only half the solution; the other half is the implementation of psychoeducational techniques to minimize, compensate for, or totally eradicate the symptoms of dyslexia. This should be our first priority, and it certainly was Sue's.

I needed to find out what Sue's problems were. I proceeded to question her about her first awareness of her difficulties.

"I was in the first grade when I experienced that dreaded disease 'school phobia.' I was unable to master the skills or the phonetics required to read. It wasn't until the sixth grade that I finally learned to read—to satisfy school requirements, not for pleasure!

"I recall I was always a poor speller and would become upset and embarrassed if I had to spell aloud. The other activity I absolutely disliked was gym because I was so uncoordinated. I remember falling off the balance beam once and feeling so humiliated. I was always the last one selected as a partner in my gym classes. Actually, whenever I played any sports or tried to perform in gym, I became physically ill and dizzy.

"I also had an auditory problem as a young child, which compounded my problems."

Sue added that she was frequently upset as a child and did not understand why she felt that way. She would pick a fight with her brother to justify her feelings. As she grew older she realized she had a severe, frustrating problem because reading was much harder for her than for her friends, especially when she had a great deal of material to read.

"I could never understand why the school could not label my problem and help me.

"Fortunately my difficulties did not interfere with me socially. I wanted very much to be a part of the group and pushed myself to participate and become involved with my friends, to convince myself and them that I wasn't different. As a result, I did not have the peer problems I sometimes encounter in my students.

"Another important factor is the support I always received from my parents. They were satisfied, and so was I, with my grades even though I was a C student."

Sue continued to find certain academic courses, such as literature and history, difficult because of the quantity of material to be read. She said she relied mainly on lectures because she was never able to complete all the readings for each college course. She even failed an art-history course because the quantity of material was overwhelming. She experienced blurring of letters and words and focusing difficulties when she read, which resulted in headaches and eye fatigue.

"Sometimes, I felt as though I were in a fog, especially in the mornings. I would find myself shaking my head, as though to clear it. The problem of concentration and being 'out of it' was more pronounced if I had a respiratory infection or an allergy attack.

"Two summers ago my reading problem was very severe. I consulted an optometrist, who prescribed glasses for my problem (poor focusing) and vision therapy. The glasses did not help much; in fact, they made me feel dizzy. But the exercises did help. Unfortunately they did not get at the heart of the problem, and I found when I was tired that the exercises did not help at all.

"My last year in college was easier because I had learned to organize my work better. I was also taking more education courses, which I found very interesting. When I read *A Solution to the Riddle Dyslexia,* I thought, This really makes sense! I knew I had to see Dr. Levinson."

Testing and consultation disclosed what Sue already knew: that she had dyslexia. She was given an appropriate program of treatment, and I asked her to record any reactions she noted and send them to me. Sue called and excitedly relayed her results.

"After only two days on medication, I was fairly sure my reading and balance were better; however, I wasn't one hundred percent sure. Within six days I was positive! Not only was my head clearer, but also letters and words were more distinct. I was reading faster with good comprehension and no fatigue and frustration.

"My balance was better. I could close my eyes and stand on one foot. I could never do that before!

"I am so excited about my reactions that I have changed the subject of my thesis; it will now deal with new theories of learning disabilities, and your hypothesis on dyslexia will head the list."

Recently, I received a letter from Sue, in which she stated: "Everything is going well. My greatly increased ability to concentrate, read, and comprehend are still with me. I finished all the required reading for all my courses this past semester—for the first time! I was even able to begin outside readings for my thesis, and I am elated. . . . For the first time I find all the reading I am doing very exciting and pleasurable.

"I no longer have a focusing problem: the vision training has become beneficial, along with the medication. During my last vision training session, to my great surprise, I was able to walk the balance beam backward! The month before I saw you, I worked on balance activities quite a lot and never got very far with them. As I told you, I never could get very far with them as a child, either.

"I was discussing with a friend, also in special education, my newfound ability to stand on one foot. I told him that now I feel that I have one focal point of gravity, at my heel, as opposed to many. In other words I had the feeling that I was being pulled from all directions. He replied, 'What you are saying is that you feel your vertical axis in relationship to your body, something we are aware that children with learning problems lack.' I found this most interesting and thought you would too.

"I have also noticed that emotionally I feel as though I am freer. I am not constantly on guard for fear that I may reveal my disabilities. I, also, feel more focused. My thoughts and actions are not as scattered as they once were. It is somewhat analogous to the sensation I feel with my balance, as previously mentioned—of having one focal point when I stand on one foot.

"My spelling, grammar, and sentence structure are also greatly improved. My mother, who has always proofread my school papers, tells me I now make very few errors in those areas. She was particularly excited after reading some pages of my thesis.

"My report would not be complete without the inclusion of my responses to an interruption of medication. Within one day after I stop taking the medication, I feel a big difference:

- The first night I have dreams of falling and of not being able to stay balanced.
- The next morning I feel 'out of it' and tend to keep feeling that way until I resume the medication three days later.
- There is no desire to read, and when I try, I have trouble tracking, even when reading just a few lines. My eyes feel as though they are pulling at each other and causing me to see double.
- I feel more unsteady.
- My old habit of head shaking to clear the fog is back.

"When I resume my medication, the positive results return: I feel great again; reading becomes easier and letters darker and sharper."

This is to be expected. I tell my patients that eventually the positive improvements will be sustained, even when off medication.* The precise time this occurs is different for each individual, but generally it is between one and four years.

Sue concluded her remarks: "I am tremendously excited, not only about my improvements via your treatment, but also about the wonderful possibilities for help that now exist for the millions of children afflicted with dyslexia and related learning disabilities."

Just prior to the publication of this book, I received the following letter from Susan, in which she enthusiastically describes her most recent improvements and how they are changing her life. I can think of no better way to summarize the phenomenon of success among dyslexics.

"I am writing this letter by hand to illustrate to you the changes in my

---

* After the first eight weeks on medication, patients go off medication on weekends and holidays to minimize development of an immunity to the drug. A more detailed explanation is found in the section dealing with treatment.

handwriting that have taken place in the last few months. There is a smoothness, evenness, and fluidity that I never had before; it is as though the writing literally flows out of my hand, although I am still holding the paper at a ninety-degree angle to my body, and am therefore writing away from myself.

"This is my last year at Bank Street School; I will be graduating in June. My last two classes are very demanding, but I am most proud to say that I am *ahead* in all the readings. As I have written before, I used to do as little reading as possible. I can't begin to describe the enjoyment I am now experiencing by participating in the class discussions of these readings.

"After a long day of teaching and as a student, I don't feel tired or overloaded. Even though my schedule is as busy as, if not busier than, it was, I seem to require less sleep—six to eight hours of sleep as opposed to ten to twelve hours I used to need. I have also noticed a change in my dream patterns and content. Previously my dreams were hectic, debilitating, and at times bizarre and fragmented. Now they are peaceful and relaxed. I think this has a lot to do with my requirement for less sleep.

"I have also noticed an interesting change with regard to my spelling. I still forget and confuse the spelling of words that were learned prior to taking my medication, but new words I have read in the literature, particularly in the last two months, I am able to correctly picture in my mind. When I became aware of this interesting phenomenon, I thought it was a fascinating concept, dealing with developmental sequences in cognitive thinking.

"I have been applying to colleges and universities for possible acceptance into a Ph.D. program in educational psychology/special education research! I never before entertained the possibility of such a venture, but now I realize that it is a possibility for me—and I am on an all-time high contemplating it.

"My excitement and enthusiasm for your theory of dyslexia has motivated me to discuss it with many people from the local school systems in my area. In fact, I will be presenting information during a few staff meetings in several districts. I have found that I receive very little criticism because I present myself as a case in point of the success of your medication treatment. I will also be discussing your theory of the inner-ear or cerebellar-vestibular system at Bank Street College during a presentation on the use of medications in special education, along with the role of the teacher.

"Additionally, I have noticed that I have developed an ability to calculate large numbers in my mind. I have always been a good math student, but I did need to work out the solution to problems on paper because I had trouble retaining the numbers and processes in my mind. However, while teaching a computer course, I became aware that I was able to calculate the solutions to problems in my mind.

"There have been so many changes in the last six months that I am truly amazed. I never considered myself impulsive, but I realize now that I was. I would be upset if I did not make quick decisions about everything, from buying a dress to deciding whether or not to take a job. I would jump into a situation or volunteer my time to a project, and then find that I did not have time in my schedule to fulfill my promise. Recently, though, I have discovered that I actually enjoy thinking about arriving at a decision—I realize that I don't have to make a split decision. I also don't feel overwhelmed when I do decide on a course of action. Finally, I feel good about my decision and don't perseverate . . . about an impulsive choice.

"Along with this loss of impulsive behavior has come the feeling of calmness, of being able to sit back and absorb what is going on without being the one always talking and monopolizing the conversation to prove that I know something. In fact, I don't think I talk as fast as I used to because I am not afraid any longer that I will forget what it is that I wish to say.

"One day, for no apparent reason, it occurred to me that I read better lying on my stomach. I mentioned this one day in class, and several people have since told me that they have had some of their students try this position with interesting success. Children who display dyslexialike symptoms tend to find this position very comfortable when reading. It seems logical that lying on one's stomach may have a harmonizing effect on the inner-ear system; it probably has something to do with the law of gravity.

"My balance and posture have improved so much that I can hardly believe it! I had always had the tendency to slouch, but I now feel as if I internally stand straight. I no longer get backaches between my shoulder blades. Also, I can walk in high-heel shoes without falling forward and looking like a klutz!

"Every day I notice something else that has changed for the better in my behavior, personality, or perception about the world. All these changes together have contributed to the wonderful feeling that I have about myself, especially these last months.

"Once again, I deeply thank you for everything."

Susan Stafford gives ample proof that one can be successful despite being dyslexic. If anything, her dyslexia has been a strong motivation in determining her goals and aspirations.

Sue had succeeded in college prior to treatment. As a result of treatment, she is completing her Master's degree with greater energy, enthusiasm, and ease than she ever thought possible. Moreover, she is now looking forward to her Ph.D., a degree she never before dreamed of attaining.

I truly believe that, one day soon, millions of dyslexics will benefit from Sue's success and contributions despite—in fact, as a result of—her dyslexia.

GARY ENGLAND

Gary England became my patient after his charming daughter, Molly, responded favorably to my recommended treatment. Gary's wife's introduction, and Gary's own description of his symptoms and responses to medication, cannot be improved upon. Here is their original content, only very slightly edited:

> After reading Gary's letter and report to you, I felt I should add some additional information. He is very modest about his accomplishments, which have been many, including "Outstanding Young Man in America." He has written two books on weather, is considered the number-one weather authority in Oklahoma, and has a higher recognition factor than the governor of Oklahoma. (Each of his books sold over 40,000 copies. . . .)
>
> In regard to the medication he is taking, the results are amazing. He also assures me that he feels better than he has in years and is so thankful to you for your research in this area. . . .

> Thanks,
> (signed)
> Mary England

Gary's report follows. . . .

"I have no recollection of specific problems in my elementary school years except that I never did well, mainly receiving C's and D's.

"During my mid-school years it was about the same. School was very difficult for me. I can recall quite vividly the frustrations of trying to do well in high school, but the results were generally still in the C and D range. I kept making the same grades as the kids who were thought to be dumb. I gave up trying to read books for book reports and reverted to using Classic Comic Books because my reading was very slow and I always had to reread each sentence to make sense. The authors' logic and word sequences always seemed jumbled to me.

"I also recall during that period a teacher saying in class that he would rather have someone who was of average intelligence who tried rather than 'Gary England, who is smart and will not try.' I believe it is very possible that my inability to make accomplishments in school is in some degree the reason that my mother said, 'Well, Gary *was* the most active of my boys.' I became rather 'wild and wooly,' as they say in western Oklahoma.

"Shortly after high school I joined the Navy. I remember that when I took a sonar test, the instructor told me I could not tell the difference between a whale and a battleship. I tried very hard to do well on the test, but it was impossible for me to determine the difference in the sonar returns from the various targets. It was overwhelmingly confusing and frustrating. Everyone around me at least scored something, but my score was a flat zero.

"My college years were a time of high hopes. However, it was a major struggle. I couldn't read well. The sentences didn't make sense. I probably studied more than most people. I seemed to have it down and then would panic during the tests and get through only the first few problems or questions. I flunked algebra and made *B*'s in higher math. I took an oral Spanish class, never understood a word, and made an *F*. However, I made an *A* in atmospheric geophysics. In the higher-level math and science courses, it seemed I could more clearly visualize what an equation or theory was all about.

"In the lower-level courses, I could never remember all the little details. During tests in those areas, it was like there was, not just a short circuit in my brain, but a total blackout.

"At one point I was taking an art-appreciation class and we were used in a research project in rote-memory learning. There was this little cylindrical tube that rotated and it had fifteen short words on it. You could only see one word at a time. As I recall, we were tested to see how long it took each student to remember all fifteen words in sequence. There were three hundred students in that class. I was the last to finish. In fact, I never really finished, as I couldn't memorize the fifteen words after two hours. Talk about frustration and feeling dumb . . . that was a low point. I finally received a Bachelor of Science degree in mathematics and meteorology in 1965.

"During the years since 1965, my wife and I have accomplished a great deal and have become what is considered quite successful. All this time I went through life feeling frustrated and fearing I was a little on the dumb side but still managing to put myself in the top-one-percent income bracket in the United States. I was not aware I had a problem other than a lack of brains.

"When someone told me a joke, I nearly always didn't understand it at the time. Later, I guess after my subconscious put the words in the proper sequence, it would pop into my conscious mind and I then would understand it. In fact, I was never very good in initial face-to-face business discussions. Much of what people said to me or plans that were laid out just did not register. The logic wasn't mine and the sequence didn't fit my sequence. However, after thinking by myself, I could sort it out until it meant something to me. Only then could I act on it and discuss it.

"I can recall, many times in recent years, reading a newspaper and discovering that a certain sentence made absolutely no sense. Some of the words were missing. I would call my wife in and, in a state of total frustration, point out to her the crazy sentence. Then, when explaining it or reading it to her, I would see all the words. This word-missing situation happened frequently when television advertisements appeared on the screen in printed form. I watched one TV station ID for several weeks before I saw the missing words. Sometimes I found that the words were there but were in the wrong place in the sequence. Brother, that is startling! I know my left and right directions. However, when driving I become lost more often than not unless I know the area exactly. Turns off of highways bring panic, and the result is that I normally take the wrong turn. To make the proper turns I have to visualize very intently the entire sequence of where I'm coming from and where I must go and integrate that with the road signs in order that the proper decision can be made. But at 55 mph, it seems there is never enough time.

"In 1975 my daughter Molly was tested and found to have symptoms of dyslexia. During a conversation with the doctor, I told him of my experiences. When I walked out of his office that day, it was like a great cloud had been lifted. I wasn't dumb, but had some of the same problems as Molly. Our conversation allowed me to realize and identify my various problem situations more rapidly. It helped a great deal to know what was going on, but it was still very frustrating to read poorly, miss words, scramble sequences, not understand what people were saying to me. I still had a poor memory, became lost while driving, and all of those other things.

"Every day I was becoming more aware of when I was having a

malfunction, so to speak. When Molly came back from the visit to your office, I was almost desperate for help.

"When you prescribed medication, I waited for instant improvement. It wasn't instant, but it began. I can really read for the first time in my life, and I have read several books. My memory—I'm telling you, it's exciting to have one now! In the past, if I attempted to remember a name from years ago or sometimes from the day before, I drew a blank. Now names pop into my mind from ten years ago.

"My memory seems to be improving daily. When I read the newspaper, the editorials make sense. When I watch television and the printed words come up, they are normally all there. I don't become lost as often while driving. Now I can sit in a business meeting, understand what is going on, and enter into active discussion. (However, my wife still says I don't hear a word she says!)

"My improvement has been significant and I really feel good about it. There are times when I still experience various dysfunctions and I find myself lost, sentences seeming to be messed up, I am unable to recall the name of a good friend, [etc.]. It is good to report, though, that such situations seem to be fewer and fewer as time goes by."

Gary is Chief Meteorologist for Oklahoma City's KWTV—a public figure who, indeed, is very successful despite dyslexia.

SULA KAUFMAN, PH.D.

Dr. Sula Kaufman, formerly a pianist and music instructor at Julliard, is currently a researcher and writer, sixty years of age and very young. She has suffered from dyslexia throughout her life. Upon examining her, I was impressed with her intelligence, perceptiveness, and charm. I asked her to record her symptoms and medication responses. Since there was no way that I could improve upon Dr. Kaufman's sincerely expressed report, I decided to present her statement just as she wrote it, with only slight modification.

"Hiding from prying eyes was the one skill I practiced to perfection during my growing years. . . . With time, it became second nature to pretend that all my difficulties were nonexistent. Perhaps it was a skill I acquired to survive, for as a child I had to cope with a condition I could not comprehend. This pretense helped me to erect a fairly positive self-image, although there is little doubt in my mind that the dysfunction must have had a dominant role in shaping my character, and was unquestionably a factor in shaping my life. . . . My childhood was filled with apprehension and terror. I knew that in certain situations I could undergo a complete change in behavior, a total metamorphosis in the way I felt. It always happened at the most unexpected and awkward moments, and I used to dread it in advance. When caught and exposed, I would stand there shaking and trembling. I also had an overwhelming fear of water and an extreme intolerance of heights.

"Being afraid of water, of course, made me afraid of swimming. I fought hard to overcome this terror: I took swimming lessons and made myself float. At times I even managed a few swimming strokes with a kind of desperate determination to overcome my absolute terror. I never could even attempt to overcome my extreme fear of heights. It used to be the only situation in which I would become nauseous and light-headed. Then, too, I always had a persistent problem with spelling, an inability to memorize the multiplication table or a simple short poem. My handwriting is often illegible even to myself—the lines are never straight and the size as well as the spacing between the letters changes twice or even three times on one page. On the other hand, I always had a very good memory for content. Although I could not memorize the multiplication table, I could always remember dates and telephone numbers, and as a student I had a good head for mathematics and languages. The contradictions did not stop there, for while I lacked the necessary balance to ride a bicycle, I was a good and agile dancer.

"My inability to memorize the multiplication table and my poor spelling seemed to me mere trifles. These were more than adequately compensated for, as I was an excellent student and an avid and voracious reader. On the one hand there was in me always an awareness that something was radically wrong with the way I functioned; on the other hand, I knew myself to be a highly capable and competent person. I always felt totally secure in some areas, while in others I was, and still am, plagued by constant devastating doubts. . . .

"I began to feel intense and persistent light-headedness combined with severe disorientation some eight years ago, after being in a car accident. Because this barrage of discomfort started soon after the accident, I did not think at the time that a connection existed between the condition responsible for my phobias, spelling, etc., and the total mess I found myself in so suddenly. The frequent X rays that were taken failed to explain or support my description of the symptoms I had. It was indicated to me more than once that my condition was largely psychological, post-

menopausal, and not atypical of hysterical and hypochondriacal women.
Had it not been for the tests given to me in your office, I probably would
have never made the connection and would have never guessed that the
accident had aggravated an existing condition.

"The sensations artificially brought on by the tests were identical in
kind and severity to the disorientation and light-headedness I lived with
for the longest time after the accident. They affected my capacity to think
as my mental process became enveloped as if by haze or fog; to top it
off, I also became markedly aphasic, and the slightest turn of my head
used to bring on severe dizziness. I fell repeatedly for no apparent reason.
At night my bed became a heaving, slanting surface; the sensation of
sliding down to the floor was so strong that I used to hold on to prevent
it.

"During that period I was also subject to fainting spells. Driving was
a problem; going in reverse was particularly impossible. But most difficult
of all was the abrupt change in life-style—from a very active one I found
myself steadily gliding into a deteriorating one.

"Eventually, however, my condition did stabilize to the point that I
could function selectively.

"I must hasten to tell you that only one drug you prescribed for me
gave me tremendous relief; with another there was an immediate excessive
weakness, including chest pains and continuous cold sweat. A third drug
had neither a positive nor a negative effect on this aspect of my functioning. The effective drug also had a fantastic effect on me in other
ways. Never in my life did I feel as well as I did when taking it: I had
boundless energy, but what pleased me most was that it was not euphoric;
rather, anything and everything I did was done effortlessly and with gusto.
Most of all, I enjoyed a feeling of being enormously alive. The only
negative effect it had was that I started driving much too fast and had to
slow down a bit. Another thing was that all through that time, I got up
in the morning feeling rested, wide awake, and ready for action. What
a contrast it was with my lifelong feeling of morning fatigue. The fly in
the ointment was that I started 'ballooning'—the weight gain in those
few short weeks was considerable.

"Perhaps I should tell you about how well I felt for the duration of the
medication therapy. Indeed, I do retain the memory of how good it feels
to be functioning fully. There was a kind of quiet uninterrupted flow of
energy I had always hoped to have. In my former 'normal' state of being,
in order to accomplish anything, I must exercise determination, self-
discipline, and willpower, and in addition I must impose upon myself an

external regimen carefully monitored by a rigid schedule. In this state there is always a sensation of a real physical barrier between volition and completion of a task, whereas the effect of the medicine allowed the two parts [to flow together].

Dr. Kaufman described her feelings further in a telephone conversation:

"I am no longer afraid to admit I lacked something, but I first needed to overcome an emotional resistance. My spelling, always poor, never really bothered me. My physical disabilities, such as lack of balance, were terrible. I could not walk a narrow path; it was not a question of fear— I simply could not walk. The whole world turned upside down for me. I felt ill and I would begin to tremble. I lost my sense of dignity.

"I never did feel stupid though. I felt different. I never encountered any one person who acted or felt the way I did, or had a selective inability to function in certain areas.

"There were numerous men who told me I was beautiful. I think I flirted and courted those compliments because it was the only way to confirm to myself that I was beautiful and not ugly. I felt as though my hands did not go with my body. It was terrible. Only when I was dancing did I feel total and beautiful. I even used to nag my husband to tell me I was beautiful. Not that he did not say it voluntarily; it was just that I had a need, a craving, to confirm my existence.

"You can not imagine how excessive my need was to do well academically. It was more than a simple need to achieve: It was a vital necessity to counteract my disability.

"I have not played the piano lately because my disability has worsened in recent years. It used to be that on a bad day I would lose the feeling in my left hand. I could not concentrate on both hands. When you play the piano, you use both hands but you look at the middle of the keyboard; you are aware of the periphery. But I could not see the periphery—I could not even look for the periphery. I would lose my place and it shook me up terribly. I did not know what I was doing.

"Another strange phenomenon would occur: I would be playing quite fluently, and suddenly I wouldn't be able to move my hands; the motion would be gone and my fingers would become quite stiff. I had been told I had arthritis in my hands and that that was the reason for the loss of motion and stiffness. But that was not so. It was as though my hands and my mind were two separate beings without direct communication.

"The medication you prescribed was amazing. Previously my playing would fluctuate, especially in the last few years. . . . After taking the medication the first time, I selected a complicated piece and began to play. I was astounded at how well I did. I was functioning in a fluid style. I acted automatically. I did not have to think, I must do this now and next I must do that, etc. I felt my hands were truly mine, acting in unison with my wishes, doing what I wanted them to do.

"The only functions that seem to be unaffected by the medication are my writing and spelling. When I write anything, I must check every other word with the dictionary. I can look up a word, write it, and then come across it on the next page, but again I must look it up.

"Dr. Levinson, I am sharing my experiences and feelings with you and your countless other patients so that they will not feel stupid anymore."

I referred Dr. Kaufman to an endocrinologist on the suspicion that she had a hidden hypothyroid disorder. Laboratory findings verified this suspicion, and she is already responding favorably to treatment.

Once again, it is crucial to note that dyslexia may coexist with other medical disorders and that the resulting symptoms may be codetermined. Thus, Dr. Kaufman's fatigue and difficulties were due to two factors requiring two different but concurrent approaches. As you may remember, my daughter Joy also was diagnosed as having dyslexia complicated by hypothyroidism.

"THE PRINCESS AND THE PEA"

Randy Martin, a dynamic female executive in her forties, was, to all outward appearances, extremely self-confident, bright, articulate, in total command of herself and her world. Inwardly, however, she was filled with anxieties, phobias, and doubts with regard to her physical and mental well-being.

As an infant, Randy suffered a severe ear infection with high temperatures.

As a young girl, she was a slow reader and experienced difficulty with spelling, math, memory-related activities, and grammar. Randy was seized by a fear of falling whenever she had to climb down stairs; she would remove her shoes in order to be sure she would not fall. Her health was complicated by a thyroid condition, and she was extremely sensitive physically. Her mother would jokingly refer to her as "the princess and the pea" because of this extreme physical sensitivity. Remarks like these, particularly from her mother, always stung.

Throughout her adult life, Randy had been motivated by a strong desire to excel and prove her worth and ability. She knew she had to work harder than others to achieve.

Randy was extremely active in a number of organizations in a variety of fields—business, the women's movements, and civic matters, such as pollution. She felt better about herself if she was very active and involved. Thus her schedule was very full and demanding. No sooner had one challenge been successfully met than she sought another. She needed to be constantly busy.

Admired and respected by colleagues and friends, Randy nevertheless could not rid herself of the feeling that she was really stupid. Even her many successes did not totally convince her. Her constant round of activities kept others from getting too close to her. She was afraid that they would find out that she had "fooled" them into thinking she was very bright and exceptionally competent.

The many physical and psychological demands placed upon Randy's time and energy produced a life-style that became more and more stressful and filled with a great deal of discomfort. Once she attended an international conference and, when she returned home, experienced "burnout"—anxietylike symptoms. She had sweaty palms, shortness of breath, feelings of faintness and of being off balance, difficulty swallowing, and the sensation of being "out of it." Although she had always loved the excitement and bustle of the city, she suddenly felt that she couldn't stand it anymore:

> I could not tolerate the city. It had become unbearably stressful for me. I couldn't breathe; there was too much movement, too much activity.
>
> I became afraid to drive and afraid to fly. I had always been an excellent driver, but now I was even more frightened to be a passenger in a car. I felt the car would fly away and crash!

Randy was scheduled to fly to San Francisco to attend an important seminar, and she was in a state of panic. She visited her physician and described her neurophysiological symptoms and phobias, explaining that she had to attend the seminar and needed help to do so. The physician had been a flight surgeon at one time, and he stated that he thought her motion phobias were suggestive of an inner-ear problem. He prescribed an antihistamine that he thought might help. She took the medication.

Randy flew to San Francisco and rented a car while she was there. While attending the conference, she read a great deal of material and participated very actively with an intellectually stimulating group. She felt fine—entirely free of symptoms.

While in San Francisco, Randy saw me on a TV program. She listened keenly to my explanation of the relationship between the inner ear and learning.

> Something clicked inside me. When I returned home, I again saw a TV rerun of the *Donahue!* in which several of your patients described their symptoms. With a burst of shock I thought, These are my symptoms these people are describing!
> Then and there I made an appointment to be examined.

Tests verified that Randy did indeed have dyslexia. In fact, special inner-ear testing (ENG) produced a precise replica of the anxiety attacks she had been experiencing on and off for many years.

When she was told the diagnosis, Randy's initial reaction was one of relief that there was something definitely wrong of a physiological nature. Therefore she was not crazy. That was an immensely profound experience for her:

> I feverently wished I could tell my mother, See, I'm not stupid. I am smart. All my life, while my mother was alive, I could never please her, never be as smart or as correct as she wanted me to be. I wanted to shout from the highest rooftop, See, I was right! Something was wrong and it wasn't my fault!

In the light of her diagnosis, Randy's fears of driving, flying, and any fast movement became understandable. For Randy everything moved five times faster than for a "normal" person. Thus, a car moving forty miles per hour appeared to be moving two hundred miles per hour. Her other neurological symptoms and difficulties also became comprehensible, including her supersensitivity. No longer did she feel in the wrong because of this body sensitivity.

Randy's second reaction to her new knowledge was anger—anger that no one had been able to diagnose her problem before. She was particularly furious with her psychoanalyst. She visited his offices:

> I yelled two thousand dollars' worth. I was livid with anger. I had been afraid to fall down the stairs because my balance and coordination was off, not because I was afraid of success. My inability to walk from one block to another at times was due to this problem of coordination and not of the mind. My fears and phobias were also related to my inner-ear disorder and not to my mind.

Randy recalled that during 1975 her life had been particularly stressful because she had been involved in very difficult and important business negotiations. She had been required to travel between Cleveland and

Detroit frequently. She was working and pushing very hard. She experienced what she called mini-seizures: faintness, difficulty in breathing and swallowing, a feeling of being off balance, etc.

> I visited a renowned neurologist and complained about these symptoms. After exhaustive tests and examinations he concluded that there was nothing wrong with me from a neuromedical viewpoint.
>
> I am furious with these so-called experts who make you feel stupid and crazy. Now I am free; I know that I am not stupid, nor am I allowing my imagination to take over.
>
> I felt a sense of great relief; over and over, the thought that I was free kept returning to me. I did not have to look for hidden, psychological meanings in my actions or feelings. I now knew that they wre physiologically based, not psychologically based, as my doctors thought and I feared.

Randy was placed on medication to help compensate for her dyslexia. She felt much better almost immediately. She is no longer taking medication on a regular basis. A virus or a toothache will trigger the dizziness, lack of coordination, or other symptoms of dyslexia. At these times she takes the medication and the symptoms are alleviated.

Randy stated that the single most important result of her visit to my offices was the realization that her lifelong difficulties and problems were of a neuromedical nature and not of her doing. She understood for the first time why her life had been such a struggle. She had achieved her goals, but with a much greater expenditure of time, energy, and effort than was required of others. With this understanding came self-acceptance.

Randy no longer feels driven to move from one activity to another, no matter how worthwhile. She is still very involved in business, civic, philanthropic, and entrepreneurial affairs, but her involvement is motivated by genuine desire, not the need to prove her intelligence. She has learned to acknowledge her brightness and no longer requires outside approval to feel successful and smart.

In all areas of her life—personal, business, and social—Randy has truly become her own person. Her pain has been lessened. She still seeks new challenges, not to prove herself, but to fulfill herself. She has learned to acknowledge her talents and to accept the fact that when difficulties occur, they have a physical basis and can be dealt with accordingly.

As a result of all she has endured, Randy has become adamant about the need for revision in our dealings with the learning-disabled. She has reiterated that her values and attitudes about herself and important others would have been different, and the course of her life altered, if her condition had been diagnosed when she was a child: Randy has been urging that neurophysiological, psychological, and educational forces combine as a single unit to deal with learning disabilities in order to help children develop self-esteem in the learning environment and to find school a positive, fulfilling experience instead of a psychologically debilitating one leading to failure and negation. She has suggested the formation of support groups to reinforce new ideas and concepts.* She believes that strengthening one's ego or self can best be achieved when people with similar disabilities assist one another to cope, to move ahead past the disabilities to reasonable success.

I agree with her! Ideas such as Randy's are valid and realistically possible if individuals who share these views work through their local communities and schools to implement them. Without implementation, such concepts are valueless.

One such support group has already been created by a large group of my Sacramento patients. They meet on a regular basis for the purpose of sharing information and experiences as well as for helping one another to better understand and deal with their or their children's dyslexic symptoms. They provide assistance and guidance in dealing with teachers, school systems, and interpersonal relations. The group publishes a newsletter from time to time, and members are happy to explain and discuss the assistance they have received at my Medical Dyslexic Treatment Center.

Randy was successful even before she knew she was dyslexic. But she is even more successful now.

* See Appendix D for more on support groups.

13
Variations of Dyslexia—With Case Histories

A CLEAR UNDERSTANDING OF THE SYMPTOMS AND MECH-
anisms defining dyslexia inevitably led to the discovery that:

- Dyslexia need not occur in "pure" form.
- Dyslexia need not be of a hereditary or congenital origin.

In other words, two more additional assumptions and convictions about
this disorder were proven to be incomplete and thus tragically misleading
to millions and millions of patients:

- Dyslexia *may* be inherited and *may* occur in "pure" form—but needn't!

By recognizing the *quality* of the symptoms and mechanisms characterizing dyslexia, it became apparent that many patients suffering from
whiplash injuries, concussions, etc., had dyslexialike symptoms. They
complained of such "psychosomatic" symptoms as blurred vision; difficulty reading because of poor tracking; concentration and memory difficulties; slurring of speech and word-finding–memory uncertainty; impaired writing and spelling; poor balance and coordination; dizziness; and
motion sickness.

Moreover young children with severe or repeated ear infections were
occasionally noted to stop talking or walking properly; some actually

became hyperactive and distractible. Early-reading children suddenly began to stumble, fumble, trip, and fall, demonstrating reading reversals and typically dyslexic tracking, memory, and concentration difficulties.

As a result of these observations, I came to the realization that these children *acquired* dyslexia in their early grades. They were not born dyslexic! Additional observations and research led me to discover that many children with mental retardation, cerebral palsy, and deafness had dyslexialike symptoms. Thus, I began to wonder:

- Is it possible that the mentally retarded, cerebral-palsied, and deaf might also be dyslexic?
- Would this assumption not account for their dyslexialike symptoms?

Prior to my research, traditional theory maintained that:

- You were either dyslexic or retarded.
- You were either dyslexic or cerebral-palsied.
- You were either dyslexic or deaf.

But this is not so! Over a period of many years I clearly proved that:

- Dyslexia may be *acquired* as a result of whiplash and concussion states as well as ear infections, mononucleosis, or any disorder affecting inner-ear functioning.
- Dyslexia may remain hidden and *mixed in* with other coexisting disease states, such as mental retardation, cerebral palsy, and nerve deafness.

In fact, dyslexics may even appear retarded and may therefore be misdiagnosed as such. I have called these cases "pseudoretarded."

These insights led me to treat these *variations* of dyslexia medically. As a result of treatment:

- *Acquired* dyslexics may suddenly be able to function more normally, return to work or school, and once again resume enjoyable, "successful" living.
- *Mixed* dyslexics suddenly blossom in their overall functioning, regardless of whether or not they have mental retardation, cerebral palsy, or nerve deafness.
- *Pseudoretarded* children suddenly appear *obviously* normal or only dyslexic.

(Reminder: No one should attempt to treat himself without consulting a doctor.)

To highlight and illustrate these observations, I will now present you with a series of recently diagnosed and treated cases—never before recognized to be dyslexic, never before believed treatable.

Acquired Dyslexia: Postconcussion Syndrome

MARY ANN ADAMS

Diagnosis: Acquired Dyslexia/Postconcussion Syndrome

Mary Ann Adams, thirty-nine, sustained a severe head injury in an automobile accident in July 1981. During the accident she struck her head on the windshield and consequently suffered a severe *organic brain syndrome*. She was referred to me by her neurologist for diagnosis and treatment.

Mary Ann was found to have exceptionally severe, magnified dyslexialike symptoms. Her speech was marked by a severe word-finding and articulation impairment as well as significant slurring and stuttering. She became unable to read: The print appeared blurry and in motion. Her writing drifted aimlessly from one side of the page to the other. Her spelling became severely impaired. Simple computations became a major burden. Her concentration and memory functions regressed, almost coming to a halt. Her balance and coordination were totally off. She could not stand alone or walk unless someone held her arm to compensate for her poor imbalance and weak muscle tone.

She became fatigued easily and suffered headaches, vertigo, and motion sickness.

She developed a multitude of phobias: She feared walking, talking, elevators, escalators, crowds, and cars. She became easily confused and panicked, blanking out, freezing, becoming what appeared to be catatonic.

Mary Ann was diagnosed to have severe impairment of her inner-ear (and cerebellar) system and was treated with a combination of medications. Within a relatively short period of time she dramatically improved. As of this date, her reading, writing, spelling, math, memory, speech, concentration, directionality, balance, and coordination are almost within normal limits. Her phobias are gone.

Mary Ann was advised to return to work six months ago. However, the telephone company refused to take her back at the time. They couldn't believe she would be able to function.

Often accident cases are thought to be malingerers who can work, but do not wish to. In this case Mary Ann *demanded* to go back to work. They refused to take her back. It took a multitude of physical examinations before she was allowed to return to her job.

She is doing exceptionally well at work now, just as she does at home.

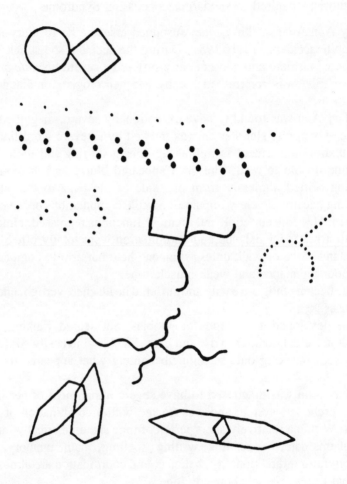

Figure A

Patients are asked to draw Figure A when they visit me for the first examination. Mary's first drawing is Figure B. After two months on medication she drew Figure C. Almost a year after her first visit, her writing and drawing were much improved (Figure D).

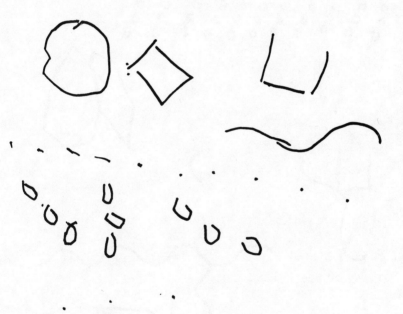

Figure B

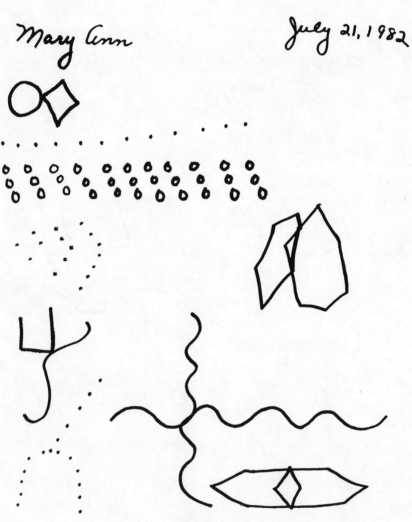

Figure C

Figure D

Acquired Dyslexia: Ear Infections

TROY DUDAS

Diagnosis: Pseudoretardation

I first examined Troy when he was six years old. He appeared to be in a fog, unable to communicate his thoughts verbally and demonstrating a significant lag in understanding my questions. He seemed retarded.

Troy had suffered from ear infections from eight months of age to four years. As a result of a severe speech articulation problem and generalized memory difficulties, Troy was tested by a psychologist in his school district. Testing revealed Troy's IQ to be normal despite low to normal scores in vocabulary, listening ability, and understanding of instructions. Many testers would have been misled by these low scores and would have misjudged him as being borderline mentally retarded or having a low normal IQ.

Three months after medical treatment Troy was psychologically reevaluated. In the doctor's report it was noted that while this growth pattern was uneven and although more complete testing was needed, there was evidence of changes in Troy's ability to attend and to concentrate. The doctor concluded that maturation alone could not account for Troy's growth in attention, concentration, auditory memory, and visual-motor integration. The doctor felt that my medication had apparently given Troy an increased awareness of his surroundings and a better ability to reflect and interact. The change was dramatic to him, since he had observed Troy's progress for over a year. In addition Troy's teacher remarked on his increased participation in class. The report concluded that readiness for learning language activities had been enhanced.

According to Troy's mother, "After only two or three weeks of treatment he began to question everything. Over the past year he has demonstrated a significant improvement in speech, awareness, memory, and behavior. . . ."

I found Troy to be a very different boy from the one I had met a year earlier. All of his difficulties have not been alleviated, but he is significantly better and happier.

I feel Troy would have benefited significantly from an early tonsilectomy, adenoidectomy, and insertion of draining tubes in his ears. These procedures would have offered him a 95-percent chance of avoiding repeated ear infections and the severe dyslexic speech and related symptoms he demonstrated.

Troy was fortunate. His parents were interested and determined. His school system was cooperative. The psychologist testing him was alert and gifted. And he responded favorably to my medical treatment. Had any one of these essential ingredients been missing, the ending could have been significantly different.

Mixed Dyslexia: Dyslexia and Decreased IQ

JOE GUST

Diagnosis: Mixed Dyslexia

Joe Gust, a sixteen-year-old student, attends an occupational high school in Michigan, a special school for the learning-disabled. Joe is neurologically impaired and has a low IQ.

Joe's parents brought him to my offices in 1982 to have him tested and evaluated. Testing revealed that Joe was a mixed dyslexic. He had an impairment within his thinking brain, affecting his IQ, mixed with dyslexia of inner-ear origin. Joe was placed on a regimen of medication to help him compensate for his dyslexic symptoms and their effect on his decreased thinking or IQ functions.

A year later Joe returned to my Medical Dyslexic Treatment Center for reevaluation. One look at Mrs. Gust's face told me that it had been a good year for Joe. Clinical examination revealed he had improved in his coordination/balance and speech.

I asked Mrs. Gust to tell me what changes she had discerned in the past year. She began: "We feel Joe's progress since he has been on medication to be very good. Joe always had a problem with coordination, and this was the first area of improvement. I noticed Joe was moving better—jumping up and down and feeling good about it.

"The next thing I noticed was that Joe was picking up books, looking through them, and even reading. This, without any urging from me. I used to ask him to read a book, but he would say, 'No, I don't wanna.' Or he would back away from me.

"I gradually became aware that Joe's memory was better. I would tell him to complete three chores before I returned home from work that evening. But he would only remember to do one. Now he remembers to do all three. Sometimes I don't even have to tell him; he does them on his own.

"Regardless of his problems, Joe has always been persistent; he's not a quitter. For example, he failed driver education, but he took it over and earned a driver's permit. When we return home, he will have his license. We are real proud of him."

I asked Mrs. Gust if Joe noticed any differences in himself.

"Well, he has told me that he feels a whole lot better about himself. Whenever we go to the store, he says, 'Let me drive, Mom, I can do it.'

"He says that he knows now that he is not dumb. He seems to have a better understanding of his problems. His outlook, in general, is good.

"Another accomplishment for Joe is that he has a paper route with seventy-five customers. Occasionally he has a little trouble with the numbers on the houses, but he is able to figure them out for himself. The first few times he did his collecting of money, my husband went with him to help. When they returned home he said that Joe did not really need his help—he had managed just fine.

"Before your treatment Joe could tell the difference between a nickel, a dime, and a quarter; but if the money was mixed together, he had to sit down and figure out which denomination was which. That is no longer necessary. He can now calculate mentally.

"At school he works in the cafeteria, taking inventory, doing the ordering, and waiting on students and faculty—and doing a good job too!"

I asked Mrs. Gust what other changes she or the teachers at Joe's school had noticed during the year.

"Joe's speech is definitely better—no stuttering or hesitation. He is calmer when he speaks and does not speak as loudly as he did. His vocabulary is better, and he appears to think before he speaks. When we discuss something, he waits to speak, as though he is thinking, and then he says what he wants to say calmly and quietly. He is more inquisitive about everything, too, wanting to know the whys and wherefores of things.

"Joe is able to express himself better. Previously, if anyone on the block teased him or called him names, he would not answer. He would keep his feelings inside. I would tell him that he did not have to accept that kind of behavior from anyone. Now he expresses his anger and even explodes from time to time when he is teased.

"In school Joe is more coordinated in sports, especially basketball. Last year it was hard for him to pass the basketball to another person without passing it to the wrong person first. This year he is able to do it correctly the first time. He also received *B*'s in volleyball, Frisbee, football, and indoor soccer.

"Joe's writing is better: His letters are even and he writes in a straight line, not all over the page. His spelling and math have also improved: He can add and subtract pretty well. Last year he just could not grasp these concepts. Now he is working on multiplication. You know, he's just blossoming daily.

"His concentration is better. There are times when he is doing something and someone will walk into the room; he'll look up just for a second and then go right back to what he was doing before, without a break in his concentration.

"The teachers are amazed at his progress. They are very pleased because he is grasping more than they had ever expected him to.

"When we returned home from New York last year, I insisted that he be placed in reading and math classes. In the reading class he jumped from second-grade level to fourth-grade level in just one year.

"You would not believe the number of people who call me from Joe's school, wanting to know your name and inquiring how we received information from you.

"His reading teacher wrote that Joe's word recognition of newly learned words was good, as was his comprehension. His left-to-right discrimination has been consistent, and he has not exhibited any reversal problems during oral reading sessions.

"Joe's attitude toward his reading lessons has been good. He seems comfortable with himself and what he is doing in reading. Joe is becoming less dependent upon continuous teacher supervision during reading instruction."

I asked Joe if he noticed any differences or changes in himself. He responded that he felt better about himself, about the things he could do now. When I asked him if he felt smarter now, he replied, "No, not yet, but I'm getting there."

Mrs. Gust continued: "Joe's improvement has been a gradual change, but I see it more and more every day, and so does everyone else. It has been the answer to our prayers and we are very, very happy. Thank you."

Joe is more in control of himself and he has a more positive self-image and attitude. Obviously he is able to perform, within his limitations—to drive a car, have a paper route, follow instructions, and complete chores at home. As a result, he has a new sense of accomplishment and purpose.

LISA GREEN

Diagnosis: Mixed Dyslexia (Mental Retardation and Dyslexia)

Lisa Green is a shy, gentle, somewhat withdrawn sixteen-year-old with a history of severe neurological impairment. Her IQ is 40. In addition, she suffers from dyslexia.

Lisa experienced the following symptoms:

- Reading—inverted letters; read on preprimer level
- Math—needed objects, such as balls, in order to add or subtract
- Spatial relations—lack of comprehension/awareness
- Sense of time/memory—unable to recall days of week, months of years; little recall for numbers
- Direction—right/left confusion
- Speech—difficulty with speaking in sentences, rarely spoke spontaneously
- Coordination/balance—very poor; unable to tie shoelaces
- Behavior—very shy, somewhat introverted; phobic about strangers; experienced highs and lows in moods.

At the time of her first visit, Lisa was diagnosed as a mixed dyslexic and was placed on medication to help compensate for her dyslexic symptoms. A revisit a year later revealed improvements in several important areas: concentration and memory, interest in reading, increase in verbalization, perception of relationships between things, recognition of signs on the highway and an ability to copy them, something she had not been able to do before.

A third visit indicated additional improvements. This update is based on my own examinations and Mrs. Green's observations:

- Reading—continues to show interest in books and reading and to improve her recognition of words
- Writing—interest in cursive writing but concentrating on printing, which has improved with respect to spacing of letters, straightness of letters/words, awareness of margins, and speed of writing
- Spelling—written recall of words much better; oral recall still not mastered
- Behavior—frustration/anxiety levels have improved, but she needs to learn to cope with situations over which she has no control; more stable moods—less highs and lows; a little more confident

- Math—ability to do simple calculations mentally, e.g., 3 + 1 = 4; awareness that she has five fingers on each hand
- Coordination—ability to tie her shoelaces
- Speech—more spontaneous; speaks more
- Sense of time/memory—much better: knowlege of days of the week and months of the year; order of items.

Lisa still needs to develop more interest in her physical appearance. Lisa's mother reported: "On the whole I am very pleased with the improvements Lisa has made and am eager to work to help her do even better."

Mixed Dyslexia: Cerebral Palsy

HOWARD STEVENS

Diagnosis: Cerebral Palsy and Dyslexia

Twenty-six-year-old Howard Stevens has cerebral palsy. His parents brought him to my offices because he suffered from dyslexialike symptoms over and above the motor-speech-coordination problems of cerebral palsy. These were reading difficulties, distractibility, a poor sense of balance, and an equally poor spatial sense.

The Stevenses tried to help Howard as much as possible at home and enrolled him in a private school. Unfortunately the school ignored the parents' observations and suggestions and concentrated on his motor difficulties. School personnel repeatedly stated that they were the experts and knew best how to deal with Howard.

It was very frustrating to his parents. Educators assumed that Howard was retarded, but his parents knew he was brilliant: At a young age, he made up his own sign language because he couldn't say words. For example, if he wanted to say apple sauce, he would pull his shirtsleeve—apple (pull) sauce. As he grew older his sign language became even more developed and ingenious. Mr. and Mrs. Stevens have a great sense of humor. They would sometimes discuss something funny and find him laughing in the next room. Howard understood their brand of humor; sometimes he would laugh before a story had been completely told. He understood and anticipated the ending.

Although they requested that Howard be thoroughly tested, his school tested him very briefly and labeled him mildly retarded. One doctor spent thirty minutes with him and said his IQ was 65 or thereabouts. They knew he was wrong.

Although initially Howard had a teacher who worked with him as his parents did, with cards, Howard's total experience with the school was bad. This one good teacher did not have the time to work with Howard because there were regular children in the class too. The following year he was placed in a class with retarded children. He knew they were retarded and he cried for a week. He was in this class for almost two years.

Then he was placed in a class for physically and otherwise handicapped children. Again it was a misplacement, because most of the children were younger. One day his parents visited the school, and instead of finding him at a typewriter practicing spelling or reading, they found him behind a screen, practicing putting on his clothes, although he dressed himself at home. And the school knew this. He had been in this class for several years.

When Howard entered junior high he was again misplaced—with a teacher supposedly qualified for teaching hearing- and physically impaired—but she was a *regular teacher,* a cold, cold person who screamed at the children and lacked understanding. The first day of school Howard stopped to touch her, a habit of his, although he held her more tightly than he should have (one of his symptoms); she yelled at him loudly and coldly, "Let go of me immediately!" There was no "Welcome to school" or even gentle admonishment.

Mrs. Stevens complained to the administration about her yelling at the children, indicating that Howard didn't respond to that treatment. They merely said that it was her method and she had to do it. That winter was difficult; Howard was subjected to much frustration. The result was that he hyperventilated.

At one point Mr. and Mrs. Stevens were told that Howard was doing beautifully. The school encouraged them to take a vacation. When they returned in ten days they received a call asking them to attend a meeting about Howard. The teacher said that Howard had done terrible things, and, as a consequence, had received "mild" punishment. She stated that he had thrown temper tantrums and during one of these episodes had broken a typewriter. What his parents did not know until years later (from a hearing-impaired girl who had been present) was that the teacher had shaken him by the hair and then pushed him into the typewriter table, knocking the typewriter over.

They were also not told that Howard had been locked in a closed room for a period of time. He had screamed and yelled to be released. These were the tantrums the teacher had referred to. In fact, the day after their return from that vacation, Howard's parents prepared to go with their son to the school because he was so upset. He was so determined not to go to school that day, he literally tore the clothes off his mother.

The school told his parents half-truths about Howard's behavior and finally suggested that he enroll in a place for the mentally impaired.

The Stevenses met with the people at the place and they were kind. They loved him because he was the only child that communicated with them. Initially he was happy with all this interested attention, but two weeks later, when his parents visited him, the light had gone out of his eyes. Suddenly, intuitively, they knew. "Howard, you pretended to be retarded to get into this place, didn't you? "Yes, I did," he answered. They brought him home.

Mr. and Mrs. Stevens heard me on TV several times, and discussed my book with Howard's teacher and several doctors. They were very impressed. One doctor had heard me speak, and he too was quite impressed with my research. He was anxious to know about their visit to me and my treatment for Howard.

They felt my success with many dyslexics would enable me to go beyond Howard's cerebral palsy symptoms . . . would allow me to see beyond the obvious and help to correct his balance and spatial difficulties. They wanted to help their son. They hoped I could help.

And so the Stevenses and Howard left my office with a program of treatment and increased hope for the future.

STELLA PETERS

Diagnosis: Mixed Dyslexia—Cerebral Palsy, Dyslexia, and Phobias

Stella, twenty-five, attractive, with a childhood history of cerebral palsy, came for medical diagnosis and treatment because of phobias and a history of dyslexialike symptoms.

In addition to her typical cerebral palsy symptoms, Stella had experienced reading, writing and spelling difficulties as a child. She continued to stutter and suffer motion sickness when riding in a car.

Within two months of treatment, Stella experienced a series of remarkable changes. She elatedly reported that her speech was so much better that she was able to speak on the telephone for the very first time in her life. Her friends are astonished at this improvement. She felt that if only she had this medication as a child, her whole life would have been completely different.

Stella feels able to communicate with the outside world without the fear of stuttering, without the anticipation of acute embarrassment. Her extreme fear of falling or being knocked over has been greatly reduced as a result of an improved sense of balance and coordination. In fact, Stella no longer feels unsure moving around at home; she feels more in control of her movements and more confident.

Stella now feels free to speak and walk. She is no longer phobic. . . . And, as a bonus, her reading, concentration, and memory have improved as well.

Stella is so thrilled with being able to use her phone and leave her home, I have found it difficult to reach her in time to finish this report properly!

LARRY MANN

Diagnosis: Mixed Dyslexia

Larry, twenty-five years old, is another example of someone who has mixed dyslexia: He has cerebral palsy and dyslexia.

Larry had speech, reading, and writing problems—he had always been slower than his peers—and his family and teachers attributed the situation to the cerebral palsy. However, Larry also had dyslexia, a fact not known until he was examined in my office.

Although it took Larry longer to work up to the medication prescribed, once he was on full dosage, the improvements became apparent:

- Larry's writing became better.
- His speech became distinct and clearer and he became better able to express himself (thinking processes show improvement).
- His fear of heights diminished: Larry could climb a ladder to put something away in the garage, something he had never done before, according to his mother.
- His reading improved, with an increase in reading speed and fewer reversals.

His mother remarked that Larry will go up the escalator now, but he still is afraid to go down. He now *wants* to go down; before, he was too panicky even to have the desire.

Larry's attitude is good; he is encouraged by the improvements. He works for a large department store, and they have promised him a permanent full-time job if he improves his writing and speaking skills. The promise of a job, the improvements brought about by the medication, and tutorial reading help are strong motivational factors in helping Larry realize his potential.

Mixed Dyslexia: Nerve Deafness

ERIN O'SULLIVAN

Diagnosis: Pseudodeafness, Pseudoretardation

As an infant, Erin O'Sullivan, now five years old, had frequent ear infections, which resulted in his spending a lot of his time at the pediatrician's office. He was on antibiotics continuously.

At eight months he was still not sleeping through the night and was exhibiting signs of insomnia due to hyperactivity. At one and a half, it was obvious to his parents that he was slower than his peers in speaking and walking. However, his parents were reassured that there was no cause for alarm. "Our pediatrician told us that if Erin was not walking by nineteen months, then he would check matters further."

Although walking by two and a half years of age, Erin did not speak at all. He even lost the few words he knew when he was one and a half. His ear infections continued and his speech appeared to get worse, suggesting a correlation between the two.

Erin's parents became increasingly concerned and consulted his pediatrician once again. This time even he became alarmed. He suddenly wanted Erin tested for hearing and speech, and suggested the possibility that draining tubes be placed in Erin's ears in order to lessen the frequency of ear infections. A complete neurological examination was also advised. The O'Sullivans were suddenly overwhelmed.

A speech and hearing evaluation found Erin to have a severe receptive and expressive language delay.

When five months pregnant with Erin's sister, Mrs. O'Sullivan was told by one of the examining doctors: "I'm sorry, but your son is deaf and should be enrolled in a special school that can deal with deafness and resulting speech disorders." He further added: "I cannot guarantee that your new baby will not be born with the same deficiencies." Moreover he advised against further testing and the insertion of the draining ear tubes, conveying an attitude of hopelessness.

Mrs. O'Sullivan dissolved into tears. She sank into despair, both for her little boy and her yet-to-be-born baby. Fortunately her maternal instincts rebelled against the doctor's advice and its unfeeling quality. She took her son to another medical center, whereupon he was diagnosed as having a hearing loss, but not a total one, and "a global developmental delay with maximum deficits in the area of language."

Despite mounting medical costs and debts, the O'Sullivans moved to another area of the state where their son could receive special speech and language therapy. At the same time, draining tubes were surgically implanted in his ears and his adenoids were removed.

They continued to search for additional answers and help. Erin was retested. His parents were told that children with the same degree of hearing loss as Erin's generally acquire speech. The fact that Erin had not done so indicated that something else was wrong, possibly an "auditory processing problem."

Following this examination, the O'Sullivans attempted to enroll Erin in a language-delayed children's program within the public school system. However, prior to admission, Erin had to take an IQ test. A test performed by a student psychologist who worked with him indicated that his IQ was 70—within the retarded range.

Mrs. O'Sullivan blew her top. She insisted that a more realistic evaluation be given by someone more experienced in dealing with deaf children. The testing resulted in an IQ of 100. Erin was then permitted to enroll in a language-delayed children's program for four-year-olds. He was also fitted with a hearing aid to help compensate for his poor auditory acuity.

Erin's parents still sought additional help. Upon reading my medical text *A Solution to the Riddle Dyslexia,* they realized that Erin's auditory discrimination difficulties might respond to my treatment. Also, they believed the disorder was caused by ear infections that impaired his inner-ear functioning. The same doctor who had advised his parents against the trip to New York now expresses great delight over the results of that visit.

When I initially examined Erin, he was extremely hyperactive and distractible, and he verbalized very little. As a result, I did not know whether Erin was mentally retarded. He was certainly dyslexic and suffered from a severe difficulty in processing auditory input. Only a successful trial on medication would determine whether or not he was retarded.

In retrospect it is obvious why Eric was thought to be deaf. He definitely had an auditory acuity problem. In addition, however, he had a severe auditory discrimination problem that compounded his inability to listen and understand speech.

According to the O'Sullivans and Erin's doctor, the boy has progressed verbally two and a half years in the last year. He has begun printing, reading, participating in sports, socializing with his peers, fighting with his sister, etc. His attention span has increased but is still short. He still becomes frustrated and is easily distracted. But again, he is much better than before.

Upon retesting Erin, his doctor found that his auditory discrimination was a year below his chronological age. There was improvement in his auditory sequential memory and his knowledge of functional use of objects. Erin also had achieved a verbal ability two years below his chronological age.

In conclusion Mrs. O'Sullivan added: "Lots of things have happened to Erin in the last year: He is in school, he has a sister at home to play with and talk with, and he is a year older and wiser . . . but I know the medication has been the answer to our prayers."

Erin has not been cured. He is being helped. He was not retarded; he just appeared to be. His specific type of dyslexia and hearing loss were caused by a series of ear infections that did not respond appropriately to antibiotics.

Erin's story illustrates why you should always seek a second or even third opinion if you are not satisfied with your first doctor's evaluation. (As you may recall, the doctor treating my daughter Joy gave me wrong advice at first, too.)

Pseudoretardation

DAVID KIM

Diagnosis: Pseudoretardation

"I am so proud of him now. . . . David is still a little bit slow, *but he is learning* and that's what is important. He can pick up a book and read it. He can write. He knows his mathematics. It is so different . . . so different. He can even listen and speak normally now."

Her eyes brimming with tears and her voice choked with emotion, David's mother happily related the progress he had made in a year and a half.

David's case is particularly significant in that he was labeled retarded by his school system. David, six years old, appeared retarded but was really dyslexic. In a sense, he suffered from the same auditory discrimination difficulties as Consuelo Brody (Chapter 7). His auditory or sound input drifted, so he experienced speech as "blurry" and thus poorly understood it. He found it difficult to impossible to answer questions in a meaningful and appropriate fashion.

When first brought to me for examination and treatment, David's symptoms were:

- Severe memory instability for seen and heard letters and words, despite the fact that his mother worked with him three hours a day
- Angled and discombobulated writing and drawing
- Poor memory retention for numbers and poor number concepts
- Memory uncertainty for sequences, e.g., days of the week, months of the year, etc.
- Poor coordination and balance and a resulting accident-proneness
- Significantly delayed and impaired speech development with a severely limited vocabulary (David began speaking words when he was three and a half years of age and sentences when four and a half.)
- Delayed or scrambled input with resulting comprehension difficulties. For example, it was necessary to repeat words and sentences several times before David understood what was said. At times one even had to point to objects before he could connect the sound with the meaning.
- Motion-related fears, e.g., fear of escalators and of heights.

As an infant of five months, David developed a severe ear infection, a temperature of 105 degrees, and a resulting seizure. From that time on his development was noted to be significantly slower than normal. He had difficulty walking, with toilet training, and with learning to identify objects.

School was a disaster; he had to repeat kindergarten. He seemed unable to learn.

According to Mrs. Kim:

His speech was very poor. He wanted to speak but he couldn't get the words out. David would want to relate a particular occurrence in school, but he was unable to make himself understood. He would break it up into pieces and we would receive the information mixed up, i.e., the end of the story first, the first part of the story in the middle, etc. We could not make sense out of what he said, and he would become very frustrated with us because we could not understand him. He wanted so badly to express himself but could not.

David was reexamined by me six months after treatment began. His mother noted that there were definitely significant and dramatic changes present:

Before, I could work with David for a week straight about a particular subject. He would have a day or two off from school, and when we returned to the point where we had left off, he would have no recollection of what we had studied together. There was nothing. It was as if his brain had lost everything. It was terrible, but I kept on trying. I had to.

Now David comes home from school, sits on the living-room floor, and begins to do his homework—without any prodding from me. Or he sits down and opens a book to read for a school assignment. Without any problems!

Reevaluation one year later revealed a continuation of David's marked improvement. His speech is now spontaneous, fluent, and in appropriate sequence. He no longer demonstrates significant memory instability for word recall. His previously severe speech input and motor output lags are hardly evident. His mother is delighted that he can converse with her about school situations such as sex, in a manner that she never dreamt possible:

His questions reflect a normal, healthy curiosity, but they floor me because they are sensible and intelligent. Previously he was unable to organize his thoughts logically and in sequence. Now he has no problems in relating events; he speaks coherently logically, and comprehensively—no small miracle!

David's balance and coordination have also significantly improved. He is able to ride a twenty-six-inch bike. He can jump—not too high, but he can jump—something he could not do before. His emotions are steadier and his ability to tolerate stress has improved. His advance has continued despite parental separation and divorce.

What would the outcome have been had David's mother not stood behind him and worked with him in a most unselfish and determined manner? What would have happened had his mother accepted the school's diagnosis that he was retarded? What happens to millions of dyslexics who are similarly misdiagnosed?

14
Summary

IN *SMART BUT FEELING DUMB,* I HAVE TRIED TO PORTRAY
the true depth and scope of dyslexia, a disorder affecting over 20 percent
of the world's population. This book was designed to capture and describe
the essence, quality, and meaning of the many and varied symptoms and
feelings characterizing and defining this previously misunderstood and
oversimplified disorder. I hope it has provided both the layman and the
clinician with the scientific insights needed to better understand and diagnose dyslexia through a holistic medical/educational approach.

This book's content and design were inspired by the emotions and
energies characterizing the struggle and determination of thousands upon
thousands of my dyslexic patients. Their energies have fueled the forces
needed for the successful completion of *Smart but Feeling Dumb* despite
my writing inexperience.

For the sake of millions of suffering dyslexics, I truly hope that I have
properly transformed the trust, efforts, and stories of my patients into a
book they can be proud of—a book and effort they well deserve.

Appendix A:

Medications and Related Chemicals in the Treatment of Dyslexia

THIS SECTION ABOUT THE MEDICATIONS USED FOR THE SUC-cessful treatment of dyslexia and related disorders has been purposely separated from the patient responses and text to emphasize a major point that cannot be sufficiently stressed: *No one should treat himself, regardless of whether medications are judged harmless and regardless of whether medications can be bought without a physician's prescription!* Only doctors are qualified to predict the benefits and/or side effects (sometimes serious) that can follow from medical use of given drugs and vitamins or any combination of vitamins, chemicals, or medications, in light of a given patient's height, weight, general physical condition, and sensitivity to chemical substances.

Therefore, *for those doctors* who may be consulted by patients who have completed this book, I will list the various chemical structures that I used in clinically determined doses and combinations during the past fifteen years in treating dyslexics, phobics, and various other behavioral, emotional, and "psychosomatic" disorders of inner-ear or cerebellar-vestibular origin.

Chemical Name	*Brand Name*
Meclizine hydrochloride	Antivert
Cyclizine hydrochloride or lactate	Marezine

209

Dimenhydrinate	Dramamine
Diphenhydramine hydrochloride	Benadryl
Promethazine	Phenergan
Scopolomine	Transderm-Scop
Hydroxyzine hydrochloride	Atarax
Methylphenidate hydrochloride	Ritalin
Dextroamphetamine sulfate	Dexedrine
Pemoline	Cylert
Pseudoephedrine hydrochloride	Sudafed
Imipramine hydrochloride	Tofranil
Amitriptyline hydrochloride	Elavil
Brompheniramine maleate	
Phenylephrine hydrochloride	Dimetapp
Phenylpropanolamine hydrochloride	
Chlorpheniramine maleate	Chlor-Trimeton
Ergoloid mesylate	Hydergine
Deanol acetamidobenzoate	Deaner

Vitamin B complex
Ginger root
Niacin
B_6
B_{12}
Lecithin or choline

Physicians and interested clinicians may further benefit from the chapters on medication in my scientific text *A Solution to the Riddle Dyslexia.*

Some of these medications were initially used because of theoretical considerations. However, clinical experience with thousands of patients over many years led me to the use of some additional substances I initially overlooked. Existing theory is often insufficient to predict a totally holistic chemical treatment plan.

Thus, for example, patient A or his parent noted learning difficulties beginning only when allergy treatment with medication X was stopped. In retrospect, it became clear that antihistamine X had unwittingly enabled patient A to compensate for his dyslexic disorder until allergy treatment stopped (the patient had been on antihistamines for a severe allergic disorder from age two to eight). This case clearly highlights the fact that the early use of medications may be helpful in preventing the dyslexic symptomatic fallout.

I eventually came to realize that although antihistamine X was sold by a drug company as an antihistamine, the same medication might also have anti–motion-sickness potency and thus could be effective for treating inner-ear disturbances. I then began testing similar antihistamines on cases not responding to the typical anti–motion-sickness medications with which I initially became familiar.

Patient B or his parent spontaneously noted that certain vitamins recommended by his pediatrician seemed to increase concentration and even improve hyperactivity. I became familiar with this effect and began to use it to my patients' advantage.

Another patient, C, researched various chemical substances tending to increase memory, concentration, and hyperactivity. Thus, I became familiar with those chemicals.

A colleague reported to me that one of his depressed patients on antidepressants suddenly noted an improvement in his reading ability. As a result, I concluded that certain antidepressants may work in a fashion similar to the antidepressants used by psychiatrists to treat activity and concentration disorders. I also realized that many of the typical antidepressants had been reported to help phobias, behavioral disorders, and bed-wetting.

Inasmuch as many individuals suffering from phobias, bed-wetting, behavioral disorders, and depression also suffer from dyslexia, it became reasonable to use antidepressants for dyslexic symptoms and evaluate their responses, especially when patients did not respond favorably to my more "traditional" pharmaceutical agents.

Parents frequently reported that sugars and dyes produced hyperactivity and distractibility in their children. As a result, I advised parents to use a specific variation of the Feingold diet and avoid *only* those dyes having an adverse effect. Any substance triggering regression was to be avoided.

I hope that the above examples will enable the reader to better understand how the list of medications and chemical substances evolved and how my treatment results increased from 50-percent effective to 75-to-80-percent effective. The crucial factor in developing a successful treatment method for dyslexics has been my ability to listen seriously to what parents and patients tell me. Unfortunately clinicians often sidestep the remarks of parents and patients, judging them as biased and failing to recognize their own biases and the resulting devastating consequences.

Appendix B:

Criticism and Its Analysis

POSITIVE RESPONSES TO MY RESEARCH ABOUND AND THUS require no further comment at this time.

Critics, however, have argued that my concepts are too simple to be true, too complicated to be understood, unproven by independent observers, and incompatible with the cortical theories of dyslexia. . . . My clinical research designs in evaluating the effects of medication on dyslexics have also been criticized for lacking "double-blind" controls.

Although I feel that any reader who has completed *A Solution to the Riddle Dyslexia* and *Smart but Feeling Dumb* is sufficiently educated to answer these critics and even analyze their motives, these critics deserve a more personal response.

My concepts are neither too simplistic nor too complicated. They are merely *realistic*. All of my concepts were derived from and are consistent with the analyses of over ten thousand dyslexic cases. All of my concepts are in harmony with:

- The known physiology of traditional neurological and mental science
- The instincts, feelings, and symptoms of *all* dyslexics
- The experience of *all* educators and clinicians who have taken the time and effort to speak meaningfully to and examine dyslexic patients
- The data of all scientists who have attempted to duplicate my results—and many have

• The observations of all scientists, clinicians, educators, and patients who have come to my Medical Dyslexic Treatment Center or followed and tested my successfully treated patients.

In fact, *all* of my neurological and physiological inner-ear clinical findings were *independently* confirmed by renowned neurological and ear, nose, and throat physicians and scientists in a "blind" and thus thoroughly unbiased fashion. It is interesting to note that the very same neurologists who examined my dyslexic patients found and reported inner-ear–related signs and symptoms 96 percent of the time. Their findings are of special significance, because these neurologists were, and probably still are, of the belief that dyslexia is of cortical origin—despite the *complete statistical absence* of cortical findings in their case reports and the rather high (96 percent) incidence of inner-ear–system signs and symptoms.

In personal correspondence Sir John Eccles, Nobel Prize laureate for his research on the cerebellum, said that he found my blurring-speed methodology and 3-D Optical Scanner "fascinating."

In a similar correspondence Drs. Christine G. Kuipers and Cornelis Weggelaar, Bureau Dijkveld, The Hague, The Netherlands, state: "We wish to thank you for your most interesting book on dyslexia. We did some experiments with an improvised form of your blurring-speed device. The results seem to confirm yours, so we intend to perfect our apparatus. . . ."

Finally, George Pavlidis, in a paper entitled "Do Eye Movements Hold the Key to Dyslexia?"* states:

Dyslexics have been found to exhibit during reading erratic eye movement (EM) patterns and characteristics, which are different from those of all other readers. The present study shows the dyslexics' erratic EMs are present not only in reading but also in the simple sequential task of trying to follow light sources, each of which is illuminated sequentially. These results could manifest a central malfunction in dyslexics, namely sequential disability and/or oculomotor malfunction.

Similar eye-movement disturbances were reported earlier by Zangwill and Blakemore.†

Do not these findings lend support to my method of diagnosis?

I did not use "double-blind" studies—sugar versus "real" pills—in my

---

* George T. Pavlidis, "Do Eye Movements Hold the Key to Dyslexia?" *Neuropsychologia* 19 (1981), pp. 57–64.
† O. L. Zangwill and C. Blakemore, "Dyslexia: Reversal of Eye Movements during Reading," *Neuropsychologia* 10 (1972), pp. 371–373.

medication studies. As stated earlier in this text, the dyslexic patients' responses to medications were so dramatic and so unexpectedly diverse, it seemed senseless to waste patients' time and suffering on sugar pills.

If only one of approximately five or six medications helped any one dyslexic patient, and if the symptoms returned when the medications were stopped or given in too low or too high doses, and if the therapeutic effect was found to be independent of the pill's color, shape, size, or expectations of patient, parent, and clinician, then it seemed reasonable to correlate my 75-to-80 percent improvement rate with a *real* medication effect despite my not using double-blind studies. Moreover sugar pills or placebos do not result in such dramatic long-lasting improvements 75 to 80 percent of the time.

Most frequently the pattern of responses obtained from patients were:

- Unanticipated by either patient, parent, or researcher
- Contrary to expectation: Individuals desiring academic improvement were disappointed to find only positive balance, coordination, and related physical changes, and the reverse.
- Improvements occurred in areas not previously known or thought of as symptoms to patients. Thus, for example, patients frequently stated: "The print is so much sharper now. I never realized my vision was blurry. My headaches and light-headedness [or fogginess] are gone. I thought that was the way everyone felt."

Every physician must at some point decide whether or not a specific medication is working on a given patient. Most often this decision is based on two crucial facts:

- What the patient says, how the patient feels, and the observations of friends and family members
- One's own clinical assessment, especially where laboratory data are not available for decision-making purposes.

How do physicians know if the medication they are using on any given patient is *really* working or not? Can they really distinguish "real" from "fake" or imaginary improvements? Do physicians perform double-blind studies—using sugar versus "real" pills—on each and every patient before making vital decisions: medication selection, dose changes, and/or medication changes when either *no* effects or side effects occur?

The answer to all of these questions is obvious: no!

Even if the medications used by physicians were initially subjected to double-blind studies, how does one really know if a "real" or "sugar" effect is currently working on any given patient?

One doesn't!

In the final analysis a physician's clinical judgment and assessment of all available data is what counts in his therapeutic decision making. This judgment is either *sound* or *not sound* and is independent of whether or not blind studies were performed years before the drug was marketed.

The majority of drugs I use are known to improve inner-ear–related symptoms: vertigo, dizziness, imbalance, motion sickness, concentration, etc. In fact, double-blind studies proved most of these drugs effective in helping these inner-ear–related symptoms long before I and many of my colleagues began using them.

Should I have begun my medication research by reinventing the wheel? Should I therefore have begun giving my inner-ear–dysfunctioning dyslexic patients sugar pills as well as "real" pills, waited three months to retest them, tried another double-blind trial if the first one did not work, and then waited another three months to retest them all over again—even before I knew clinically whether or not the medications helped such inner-ear–related dyslexic symptoms as reading, writing, and spelling?

Once I knew the medications helped dyslexics and witnessed responses similar to those you have read, should I have conducted "real" versus sugar medication trials, or should I have attempted to treat as many patients as possible as rapidly and as effectively as possible? Should I have wasted three to twelve months of a dyslexic child's life merely to "prove" what I already knew—merely to avoid criticism?

I leave it to the reader to decide.

More and more clinically minded researchers share my point of view: Often, but not always, clinical medication trials are easier and thus more rapidly and efficiently conducted. And most important, one can zero in on positive and negative medication effects; crucial insights are thus more readily seen and heard. Double-blind studies are often most helpful when the data obtained from clinical trials are uncertain.

For double-blind studies to be performed accurately, scientifically, one really must know:

- How to measure the anticipated clinical responses
- The doses and their variations needed to obtain a classical response, if one is to happen
- That patients will respond to only one of approximately five to ten medications, suggesting that the study use sequentially but "blindly" chosen chemical groupings where responses are initially negative
- That school grades do not invariably reflect improvement, i.e., many improved individuals obtain the same grades with significantly less effort
- That any one or group of the thirteen categories of functioning may improve on any given medication; therefore *all* these variables should be measured, not just reading or writing variables.

For me to have jumped into double-blind studies initially would have been a significant mistake. And I believe the same is true for all researchers who "blindly" perform traditional procedures like robots rather than like scientists.

Inasmuch as my research efforts have been:

- The first to portray truly the scope and panorama of the various symptoms and signs characterizing dyslexia
- The first leading to a successful *medical* means of accurate diagnosis, prediction and treatment, and even prevention for a disorder that completely eluded all prior traditional medical approaches
- The first to recognize that phobias and related emotional, behavioral, and "psychosomatic" symptoms may be due to the same inner-ear dysfunction creating the dyslexic symptomatic fallout
- The first to recognize the concepts of *acquired* and *mixed* dyslexia, and thus enable the mentally retarded, cerebral-palsied, deaf, and other disabled individuals to be successfully treated for their dyslexic disorders
- The first to lead to a medically based understanding of successful educational techniques, and the first to create such techniques
- The first to explain holistically and encompass *all* other theories,

it seems reasonable to ask my critics a few questions:

- If indeed my research efforts have succeeded, whereas so-called traditionally accepted techniques have led only to scientific confusion and failure, is it not possible that there may be something wrong with "traditional" methods and techniques as they have been, and are yet being, practiced?
- Have not traditional assumptions and techniques created a dyslexic riddle in which "parallels intersect and straight lines form loops"?

In conclusion I challenge my critics:

- Find me another text, scientific or popular, that can match or exceed the insights provided by my patients in *Smart but Feeling Dumb* or in my medical textbook, *A Solution to the Riddle Dyslexia*!
- Reassess the motivation for your criticism!
- For the sake of *all* dyslexics, carefully read and observe my research and duplicate it!
- Suspend judgment until you have spoken to, analyzed, diagnosed, and similarly treated thousands of dyslexics or as many dyslexics as it takes to form a sound, realistic conclusion!

Appendix C:

Otto Fenichel on Phobias

COMPARE MY REASONING AND PROPOSED MECHANISMS TO account for phobias with the following ones described by Otto Fenichel:

> Fear of high places later may be replaced by the conversion symptom of getting dizzy spells when looking down from high places. This symptom is physical expression of a mental anticipation of actual falling. . . .
>
> Fears of falling, of heights, car and railway phobias, show at first glance that they are developed in an attempt to fight pleasurable sensations connected with equilibrium stimulation. . . .
>
> Phobias of vehicles, rooted in the warding off of erogenous sensations of equilibrium and space, have definite relations to the somatic disease of seasickness. The vegetative excitements aroused by equilibrium sensations in a purely physical way have a distinct similarity to sensations of anxiety, and these excitements may have become associatively connected with "too much sexual excitation" in childhood. Neurosis and seasickness, then, may influence each other. Persons with claustrophobia and similar neuroses probably tend more toward the development of seasickness; and an occasional seasickness in a hitherto nonneurotic person may mobilize infantile anxieties and have the effect of a trauma reactivating the memory of a primal scene. There are also conversion hysterias which are an elaboration of vehicle phobias in the sense that vomiting or dizziness, as a physical anticipation of feared equilibrium sensations, may have supplanted the anxiety.*

* Otto Fenichel, *Psychoanalytic Theory of Neurosis,* New York: W. W. Norton & Co., pp. 197, 202–203.

Appendix D:

Responses to Medication

Reading Activity
  Increased spontaneous reading activity
  Diminished dysmetric tracking and finger pointing
  Improved fixation ability
  Improved foreground-background differentiation (i.e., decreased blurring
    and increase in degree of letter blackness)
  Decreased or eliminated reading reversals
  Increased reading speed and accuracy
  Increased interest in reading
Writing Activity
  Increased spontaneous writing activity
  Smoother rhythm and increased legibility
  Improved spacing between letters and words
  Increased horizontality in writing
  Increased use of cursive writing (printing usually easier)
  Decreased writing reversals
  Increased use of grammatical details (i.e., periods, commas, etc.)
  Increased writing speed
  Increased word content
  Decreased number of spelling errors

Spelling
  Increased spelling recall and decreased letter reversals (i.e., insertion and
    omissions)
Arithmetic
  Increased mechanical alignment
  Increased memory for calculations
Directionality, Spatial Organization, and Planning
  Increased right-left differentiation
  Decreased rotations
  Increased detail in drawing
  Improvements in *Goodenough* figure drawings
  Improved spacing in writing
  Improved relationships to spatial coordination tasks (i.e., ball playing,
    catching, throwing, batting, etc.)
  Increased ability to tie shoelaces, etc.
Balance and Coordination
  Increased ability to ride a bike, dribble a basketball, etc.
  Decreased clumsiness (i.e., tripping, falling, and various postpointing and
    prepointing activities)
  Increased feeling of internal steadiness
Foreground-Background Activity (Sensory)
  Increased foreground clarity
  Improved background suppression of irrelevant and distracting events (i.e.,
    visual, acoustic, etc.)
  Decreased acoustical blurring and scrambling
Speech
  Increased spontaneity of speech
  Decreased slurring, where present
  Increased rate and improved rhythm of speech
  Increased verbal content
  Decreased stuttering, stammering, and hesitations
Sequence Activity and Memory
  Increase in sequence memory (i.e., days of the week, months of the year,
    spelling, multiplication, etc.)
Time Sense
  Increased sense of time and time sequences
Concentration and State of Consciousness
  Improved and increased clarity of consciousness and associated improve-
    ment in memory

Mood

Improved and increased stability of mood

Self-Image

Decreased feelings of inferiority and stupidity

Decreased defensive attitude

Increased self-assertiveness

Increased positive attitude

Body Image

Improved, as reflected in *Goodenough* figure drawings, and generalized sensorimotor activity

Improved visual, acoustic, tactile, temperature, olfactory, and proprioceptive modulation

Frustration Tolerance

Increased frustration tolerance

Increased concentration and attention span

Anxiety Tolerance

Increased anxiety tolerance

Socialization

Increased and improved socialization, especially with peers

Acceptance of Symptoms

Decreased denial

Increased ability to tackle, understand, and accept symptoms

Increased ability to ask questions spontaneously

Dysmetric Dyslexic and Dyspraxic Phobias, Inhibitions, Counterphobias, Characterological Development

Improved

Appendix E:

Support Groups for Dyslexics

IN SACRAMENTO, CALIFORNIA, A SELF-HELP GROUP HAS BEEN formed for families of dyslexics and for dyslexics themselves to talk about this most frustrating disorder. All the people involved in establishing this group are very enthusiastic about its success and are eager to see other, similar groups develop in other cities. (In Sacramento, contact Ed and Jackie Linn, 1211 Arroyo Grande Drive, Sacramento, CA 95825; or Don and Darilyn Thaden, 3131 Claridge Way, Sacramento, CA 95821; or Mary Torgenson, 3125 Root Avenue, Carmichael, CA 95608.)

I, too, hope that other dyslexic self-help groups develop by the end of the year. I plan to train other doctors and technicians to set up medical dyslexia treatment centers similar to my own. Once this is done, these centers will be able to work with the local support groups and school districts, so that the medical *and* emotional *and* educational needs of dyslexics everywhere will be served.

Bibliography

Adrian, E. D. "Afferent Areas in the Cerebellum Connected with the Limbs." *Brain* 66 (1943), pp. 289–315.

Dow, R. S., and R. Anderson. "Cerebellar Action Potentials in Response to Stimulation of Proprioceptors and Exteroceptors in the Rat." *Journal of Neurophysiology* 5 (1942), pp. 363–371.

Eccles, J. C. "The Cerebellum as a Computer: Patterns in Space and Time." *Journal of Physiology* 229 (1973), pp. 1–32.

Ente, Gerald, M.D. "Ask the Doctor." Nassau County, New York, Chapter of the Association for Children with Learning Disabilities *Newsletter* 1:1 (Dec. 1982–Jan. 1983), p. 4.

Feingold, Helene, and Ben Feingold. *The Feingold Cookbook for Hyperactive Children and Others with Problems Associated with Food Additives and Salicylates.* New York: Random House, 1979.

The FCLD Guide for Parents of Children with Learning Disabilities. Created and published for The Foundation for Children with Learning Disabilities (FCLD), New York, by Educational Systems, Inc., 1984 (ISBN O-931112-01-X).

Galaburda, Dr. Albert, and Dr. Thomas Kemper. "Cytoarchitectonic Abnormalities in Developmental Dyslexia: A Case Study." *Annals of Neurology* 6 (1979), pp. 94–100.

Gelb, Harold. *Clinical Management of Head, Neck, and TMJ Pain and Dysfunction.* Philadelphia: W. B. Saunders, 1977.

Koestler, Arthur. *The Ghost in the Machine.* New York: Macmillan, 1968.

Kohen-Raz, R. "Developmental Patterns of Static Balance Ability and Their Relation to Cognitive School Readiness." *Pediatrics* 46 (August 1970), pp. 276–284.

———. "Postural Control and Learning Disabilities." *Early Child Development and Care* 7 (1981), pp. 329–352.

Kohen-Raz, R., and E. Hiriartborde. "Some Observations on Tetra-ataxiametric Patterns of Static Balance and Their Relation to Mental and Scholastic Achievements." *Perceptual and Motor Skills* 48 (1979), pp. 871–890.

Levinson, Harold N. *A Solution to the Riddle Dyslexia.* New York: Springer-Verlag, 1980.

Orton, S. P. *Reading, Writing and Speech Problems in Children.* New York: W. W. Norton, 1937.

Orton, S. P. "Discussion of a Paper by Dr. J. G. Lynn, *Archives of Neurology and Psychiatry* 47 (1942) p. 1064.

Pavlidis, George T. "Do Eye Movements Hold the Key to Dyslexia?" *Neuropsychologia* 19 (1981), pp. 57–64.

Rubin, Nancy. "Wen Smart Kids Cant Lern." *Ladies' Home Journal* 101:2 (Feb. 1984), p. 66.

Snider, R. "The Cerebellum." *Scientific American* 174 (1958), pp. 84–90.

———. "Cerebro-Cerebellar Relationships in the Monkey." *Journal of Neurophysiology* 15 (1952), pp. 27–40.

Snider, R. S. "Recent Contributions to the Anatomy and Physiology of the Cerebellum." *Archives of Neurology and Psychiatry* 64 (1950), pp. 196–219.

Snider, R. S., and A. Stowell. "Evidence of a Projection of the Optic System to the Cerebellum." *Anatomical Record* 82 (1942), pp. 448–449.

———. "Evidence of a Representation of Tactile Sensibility in the Cerebellum of a Cat." *Federation Proceedings* 1 (1942), p. 82.

———. "Receiving Areas of the Tactile, Auditory and Visual Systems in the Cerebellum." *Journal of Neurophysiology* 7 (1944), pp. 331–357.

Zangwill, O. L., and C. Blakemore. "Dyslexia: Reversal of Eye Movements during Reading." *Neuropsychologia* 10 (1972) pp. 371–373.

INDEX

A

Academic performance, dyslexia and, xvi, 7, 10, 20, 56–59, 70, 82–83, 182
  dyslexic athletes in training and, 28
  in high school and college, 114
  medication and, 39, 42–43, 45–46, 47, 48, 49–50, 51, 52
  motor exercises and, 27–28
Activity abnormalities. *See* Hyperactivity; Impulsiveness, dyslexia and; Overactivity
Adams, Mary Ann, 189–194
Adaptation, dyslexia and, 27–28
  See also Compensatory devices
Adelphi University, Learning Disability Unit of, 82
Adenoids, 17
Adrian, E.D., 96
Age, medication dosages and, 35
Aggressiveness, 14
  See also Behavior problems
Agoraphobia, dyslexia and, 21, 141

Alexia, compared with dyslexia, 99–100
Allergies, dyslexia and, 26–27, 42, 101
Anderson, R., 96
Anger, 8
  See also Temper tantrums, dyslexia and
Anti-motion sickness medications, 35
  reasons for successful use in dyslexia therapy, 26
  tests with, 95–96
  See also Medication for dyslexia
Antidepressants, 34
  first use in dyslexia, 211
  phobias and, 137
  See also Medication for dyslexia
Antihistamines
  dyslexia, deafness and, 79
  dyslexia therapy and, 34, 35
  See also Medication for dyslexia
Anxiety tolerance, medication and, 220
Aphasia, dyslexic speech difficulties misdiagnosed as, 15

225

Smart But Feeling Dumb

is also available in audio cassette. The audio version is especially geared to those people who have difficulty in reading or who cannot see.

For further information, please write:

The Medical Dyslexic Treatment Center
600 Northern Blvd.
Lake Success, NY 11021